Praise for *The Ventilator Project*

'A must-read for all, particularly people associated with the government. It is a positive story emerging out of an otherwise gloomy backdrop . . . a riveting story of aspirational India. This compelling narrative outlines how if all the stakeholders – academic institutions, young startups, corporates and business leaders, the government – work together with a sense of purpose, seemingly impossible tasks can be achieved with elan. The protagonists – the members of the Nocca Robotics team – will be remembered as role models for young aspiring tech wizards from around the world. Government leaders will realize how a supportive government machinery can make the seemingly impossible happen. Corporate leaders will uncover a new purpose and their role in building a new India.

It is a story of grit, determination and sheer brilliance displayed by a young group of engineers. The authors redefine the roles of academic institutions, leaders of the government and corporate businesses in building the new India'

K. VijayRaghavan, Principal Scientific Adviser to the Government of India

'Covid has dramatically forced a pace of change and innovation in every conceivable area. Whether it is finding new markets, new ways of serving customers, building new products, reimagining supply chains or collaborating with ecosystems in new ways, every rule in the book has had to be questioned. So, this brilliantly written book is very timely. I believe this story will serve as an inspiration to challenge our own mental models and embrace a world full of opportunity and change'

Gopal Vittal, Managing Director and CEO, Bharti Airtel (India and South Asia)

'Srikant and Amitabha weave together an inspiring story that showcases how some of India's burning problems can be solved when passionate and diverse groups of people come together to create magic. They chronicle a successful (in this case, but usually elusive) academia–industry collaboration between India's science and technology institutions, startups and industry leaders. Their biggest contribution is to demonstrate how to get things done in India, especially in a rapidly changing and increasingly complex world. If such a trial-by-fire project can succeed in the midst of a pandemic, then we have reason to be optimistic about India's future'

Pramath Raj Sinha, founder and Chairman, Harappa Education; founder and Trustee, Ashoka University

'You have read about "Make in India" but this book tells the story of "How it can be done in India" (or indeed anywhere in the new connected world). The inside story of the race to produce a world-class life-saving product in the face of the Covid-19 crisis reads like a *Mission Impossible* script'

Samir C. Arora, Founder, Helios Capital Management Singapore

'The IIT Kanpur Ventilator Project will be embedded in the history of the institution for the extraordinary effort of twenty brilliant minds who rose to the occasion with innovative capability, unparalleled agility and determination to give to the country a much-needed offering to save lives in these trying times. The impossible task of designing, clinically testing and commencing production in a record ninety days stands testimony to the talent of the outstanding people who grace the hallowed portals of IIT-K. Kudos to Srikant and Amitabha for co-authoring a book to share this exemplary feat. It records for posterity a shining model of India's intellectual capacity and spirit of enterprise that will serve as an inspiration for future generations'

Sanjiv Puri, Chairman, ITC Limited

'What's the secret sauce behind creating an innovative, affordable and good-value product under the most challenging market conditions? Tech knowhow and experience, innovative thinking, rapid prototyping, accessing networks for expertise as well as funding. How these elements synthesize for a rapid turnaround from design to launch, the book tells it like it is. A fascinating read about how young innovators applied design thinking and were scaffolded towards success'

Ramesh Ramadurai, Managing Director, 3M India Ltd

'What a compelling picture Srikant and Amitabha paint, taking us through a ninety-day rollercoaster to build a ventilator, but skilfully jumping between that experience and the larger lessons for the emerging post-pandemic world. If you like jump discontinuities, you will enjoy this book. If you don't, you still must read it'

Suresh Shankar, founder, Crayon Data; President, IIMPACT (Pan-IIM Alumni), Singapore

'If you want to learn how to succeed in business, with mission over capital, collaboration over control, this real-life story is a great read. Srikant and Amitabha tell a fascinating story of facilitating 10X innovation, building a world-class ventilator at a fraction of what one assumes is the necessary cost and time. I have seen up close many small businesses rise and quickly adapt to the post-Covid world. What caught my eye in this enterprise was the brilliant way in which radical thinking, technology and tenacity worked in a physical and virtual world to beat the same odds'

Dinesh Agarwal, Founder and CEO, IndiaMART

'In Albert Einstein's words, "Only in times of crisis do great minds arise." The IIT Kanpur Ventilator Project is a true coming together of great minds and mentors. Inspiring, captivating and proving what is possible when will and wisdom come together. I hope this example of entrepreneurial spirit, innovation, the great tradition of mentorship and collaboration paves the way for pathbreaking work as an outcome of the journey so well captured in the book'

Geetika Dayal, Executive Director, TiE Delhi-NCR

'We all understand the value and importance of innovation. The extraordinary world we now live in, thanks to the Covid-19 pandemic, has eloquently informed us that it is no longer adequate to be able to innovate but also be able to do so at warp speed! Because your company, even human lives, could depend on it. *The Ventilator Project* is a wholesome illustration of the same. The book reads like a Hollywood thriller – almost like the script of *Ocean's Eleven* – where a group of twenty people, with disparate skills and expertise, residing in India and overseas, young and experienced, banded and bonded together, for a time-sensitive, seemingly impossible mission. It also reads like a management treatise about how organizations will need to increasingly operate in "any normal": embrace radical collaboration, do inventive problem-solving and operate with extreme agility. Kudos to Srikant Sastri and Amitabha Bandyopadhyay and thank you for saving lives'

Navyug Mohnot, Founder and CEO,
QAI Global Services; founder, QGLUE

'India's problems have been and will be solved by Indians. If we look at the history of the political economy, champions have come forward to create Indian solutions for India. Srikant Sastri and Amitabha Bandyopadhyay's book is a superbly articulated template which includes a toolkit for new-age innovation and entrepreneurship, making it a must-read for innovators and policy makers. It illustrates that India's many challenges are the opportunities which must be leveraged. The scale of India's complexities and many asymmetries are daunting but enable innovators to take their model to any part of the world'

Shankkar Aiyar, political economy analyst and author of
Accidental India and *Aadhaar: A Biometric History of India's 12-Digit Revolution*

'The authors tell the uplifting story of innovation, collaboration and entrepreneurship to launch a world-class ventilator at low cost in a record time of ninety days during the first months of the Covid-19 pandemic. This story of a young robotics firm applying its talent and skills to seize the opportunity to serve an urgent and immediate need exemplifies the potential of "Atmanirbharta". As mentors for this new venture, Sastri and Bandyopadhyay are inspired and inspiring. A great read!'

Anju Seth, Director, IIM Calcutta

'How do you innovate when you are facing a global crisis? Srikant Sastri and Amitabha Bandyopadhyay present the inspiring tale of how a world-class ventilator was developed in record time at IIT Kanpur. This book is a terrific read for all, including design engineers, entrepreneurs, academics, students and public-policy officials. Sastri, an IIT graduate and a proven entrepreneur and Bandyopadhyay, an eminently qualified bio-scientist, bring their gripping story alive with their narrative. The book is full of valuable lessons offered through a black-swan pandemic that calls for out-of-the-box solutions'

Venky Shankar, Professor and Coleman Chair in Marketing and
Director of Research, Center for Retailing Studies,
Mays Business School, Texas A&M University

'The ventilator design concept to commercial product in under a one-quarter period is a home-run success story of students, inventors, mentors, fund managers and doctors seamlessly collaborating to launch a much-needed medical device as the Covid-19 pandemic was beginning to peak. Groups which traditionally operated in pigeon-hole compartments united seamlessly to play the relay race in perfect synchronicity with Srikant and Amitabha as the symphony maestros. This first-of-its-kind model story will set a benchmark for entrepreneurs similar to what movies like *Lagaan* and *Chak De India* achieved in terms of sports team spirit'

Ashwini Kumar Nangia, former Director,
CSIR-National Chemical Laboratory

'Has a PVC or MVC ever been awarded to a battalion or an entire regiment? I feel that the three pillars of individuals in this book by Srikant and Amitabha qualify. While not in the armed forces, their service to the nation is a story of incredible courage. It is a story of relentless effort in the face of adversity against an enemy, in this instance invisible. Theirs is a story of sustained action beyond the call of duty. The authors are not just narrators of the story but active participants in the ninety-day event which will be written in the fabric of the nation's history. The story of these men and women is worthy of the highest bravery award'

Dr Ashish Diwan, Director, Spine Service, St George &
Sutherland Clinical School, University of New South Wales

'*The Ventilator Project* brings the much-needed focus on healthcare in India, and especially the crying need for a domestic medical equipment industry. Srikant and Amitabha have beautifully described why the medical fraternity has been sceptical about buying locally made equipment, and suggested ways to overcome this mental block. Their book shows how collaboration between doctors, innovators and scientists can be transformative. If medical tourists can come to India for high-quality healthcare, there is no reason why high-quality medical equipment cannot be produced and exported. Food for thought!'

Dr Gourdas Choudhuri, Director and Head, Department of
Gastroenterology and Hepato-Biliary Sciences,
Fortis Medical Research Institute (FMRI)

‘One book that will stand out in 2021 is *The Ventilator Project*. A timely and riveting read, a fascinating story that no one should miss out on in order to get inspired and take pride in being Indian’

Amith Prabhu, Founder and Communication Catalyst, The Promise Foundation

‘There are three types of innovation: incremental, step change and breakthrough. And ultimate breakthrough is not just about the product but about a radically new business model. *The Ventilator Project* is a fascinating chronicle of one such ultimate breakthrough. It exemplifies how businesses can succeed at the speed of light in this new world. It has lessons not just for India but for Silicon Valley and the world. The authors bring this fascinating story to life while distilling the lessons and key steps to replicate breakthrough innovation in your business’

Kandy Anand, CEO, Igniting Business Growth LLC

With a blueprint for business in the post-Covid world

the Ventilator Project

How the IIT Kanpur Consortium Built a World-class Product during India's Covid-19 Lockdown

Srikant Sastri and
Amitabha Bandyopadhyay

MACMILLAN

First published 2021 by Macmillan
an imprint of Pan Macmillan Publishing India Private Limited
707, Kailash Building
26 K. G. Marg, New Delhi - 110001
www.panmacmillan.co.in

Pan Macmillan, 6 Briset St, Farringdon London EC1M 5NR
Associated companies throughout the world
www.panmacmillan.com

ISBN 978-93-89104-66-0

1 3 5 7 9 8 6 4 2

Typeset in Sabon Roman by SÜRYA, New Delhi
Printed and bound in India by Replika Press Pvt. Ltd.

To our fellow Indians for their collaborative and fighting spirit during the pandemic, especially the frontline warriors

&

To that great institution, IIT Kanpur, which has given us both so much

Contents

Foreword

The Covid-19 pandemic has caused havoc throughout the world. At the time of writing, India is one of the most severely affected countries. The pandemic has also led to widespread economic disruptions, plunging the country into recession. The silver lining, however, has been that it has fuelled several innovations and startups within a short span of time and created new opportunities for many entrepreneurs.

When the pandemic first struck India in early March 2020, it was predicted that the country would soon have to face an unprecedented crisis if immediate steps were not undertaken. From inadequate healthcare facilities to non-availability of testing kits and labs, protective equipment, such as PPE kits and N95 masks, and advanced medical equipment such as ventilators, India looked completely unprepared to face the enormity of the crisis. On 23 March 2020, Prime Minister Narendra Modi declared a nationwide lockdown to halt the progress of the disease in the country. The Government of India swiftly put into action a comprehensive plan for preparing the healthcare system of the country to face the impending crisis. The government's action in part galvanized the entrepreneurial ecosystem of the country. Industrialists and entrepreneurs seized the opportunity that the crisis ironically offered, and, within a short time, India set up several enterprises that not only produced N95 masks, PPE kits and other products to meet our requirements but even started to export them globally.

IIT Kanpur has had a long tradition of innovations and incubation. Recently, we have consolidated all the activities of the incubator under a Section 8 company called Foundation for Innovation and Research in Science and Technology (FIRST). FIRST is popularly branded as Startup Incubation and Innovation Centre (SIIC), which is professionally managed by its CEO, Dr Nikhil Agarwal, under the overall guidance of Professor Amitabha Bandyopadhyay (one of the authors of this book). We are also very fortunate to have an eminent board with Dr Saurabh Srivastava, Mr Srikant Sastri (the other author of this book) and Mr Manoj Kumar as its members. With renewed thrust on incubation activities including faculty entrepreneurship policy for commercialization of research being undertaken at IIT Kanpur, many innovative enterprises have been incubated here in the last couple of years. With more than seventy-five companies currently being incubated in diverse areas such as agriculture, aviation, education, healthcare and biotech, water and sanitation, and social enterprises, SIIC has created an impressive portfolio of dedicated and passionate entrepreneurs. SIIC offers mentoring by corporate leaders of national and global business organizations, support for legal and intellectual property rights, and above all, helps build connections with leading angel investors and venture capitalists.

With such a rich ecosystem, it was natural that IIT Kanpur should rise to the challenge thrown by the Covid-19 crisis. Under the dynamic leadership of Professor Bandyopadhyay, several project ideas were floated to incubated companies. I was pleasantly surprised that many faculty members also responded to the call and took up several challenging research and development (R&D) projects that included the development of a disinfectant chamber, a positive pressure respiratory system, PPE kits, oxygen concentrator, nano-fibre-based N95 masks, protective surface coating for N95 masks and more!

However, the idea of developing an indigenous invasive ICU ventilator was one of the most challenging of its missions. Given the fact that an ICU ventilator is a complex medical device that requires high precision of operation by trained specialists in a critical-care setting at a hospital, it was almost certain that even if the IIT Kanpur team developed the technology, the final product would become available only long after the pandemic was over.

But responding to the institute's call, the Nocca Robotics team decided to take up the challenge. Incubated in IIT Kanpur in 2017, Nocca Robotics had been developing an autonomous and waterless solar-panel-cleaning robot. A task force with some illustrious IIT Kanpur alumni and other eminent experts was set up in March. Within ninety days, the impossible was achieved. A world-class ventilator with many advanced features, and Internet of Things (IoT)-enabled control was being tested in an ICU setting by intensivists after less than three months of intense efforts, during a most difficult period when the entire country and the world were under lockdown. The team also received immense cooperation from several central and state government ministries and agencies. Pune city officials enabled the team to work during the lockdown. The Ministry of Electronics and Information Technology and the Cabinet Secretariat of the Government of India acted on our request and helped with the sourcing of components. It is truly amazing how this feat was accomplished in a record time frame. This book narrates this extraordinarily inspiring journey.

This is not just a story of innovation or product development by an IIT Kanpur startup or one about amazing teamwork. This is also a story of dedication, passion, commitment, collaboration, coordination and, above all, patience. This is an account of how a team of global corporate leaders, experienced medical professionals, scientists from IITs, young, budding engineers and entrepreneurs living and working in different parts of the country came together to produce a state-of-the-art medical device in adverse working conditions.

Our prime minister has articulated his vision of 'Atmanirbhar Bharat'. The primary intent behind the vision is that as economic activities grow in India, we should reduce our dependence on imports. Globally, nations are increasingly becoming aware of intellectual property rights (IPR) and using IPR reserves to position their international trade policy. Self-reliance in technology is also needed for strategic and national security reasons. This has been witnessed in the wireless communications industry, where, during the second and third generation (2G and 3G) phase of communications systems, most of the IPRs were held by Western nations. But a greater ownership of IPR in the fourth and fifth generations (4G and 5G) has shifted to Asia-Pacific countries. India still has negligible contributions with respect to IPR, despite being the second-largest telecom market in the world.

The critical elements for the success of 'Atmanirbhar Bharat' and the 'Make in India' missions are design and IPR creation leading to product manufacturing. Academia can play a significant role in driving innovations, creating intellectual property, incubating startups and contributing to global standards with standards-essential patents. Indian academia has significant potential. However, most of it is primarily focused on R&D towards publications. We need an increased emphasis on translational research driving innovations. For our country to design, develop, manufacture and commercialize globally competitive products, we need close linkages between translational research in academia and industry. The Government of India's vision of setting up technology business incubators and university research parks on the campuses of academic institutions where industry R&D personnel and entrepreneurs can closely work with faculty members is a step towards enhancing such collaborations. We need to create a sustainable and thriving innovation ecosystem of startups and an R&D-driven industry that can harness the potential of our young graduates.

The story of the IIT Kanpur ventilator demonstrates that the youth's talents, energy and enthusiasm, when guided and channelized by experienced leaders, can do wonders. It has shown how academia can play the role of a catalyst in building affordable state-of-the-art technology. It has shown how close collaboration between industry and academia can drive an innovative and globally competitive product. I hope this book will inspire our academicians, entrepreneurs and industrialists to collaborate more closely to help India become a leader in technology development.

Abhay Karandikar
Director, IIT Kanpur
16 December 2020

Preface

8 August 2020

It was a normal working day at the ICU of Ruby Hall Clinic, Pune, though as normal as it could be during Covid times.

A patient in respiratory distress was being shifted to the unit from another hospital. Breathing through an NIV (non-invasive ventilator), she was desaturating rapidly in the ambulance. The ER staff insisted that she needed urgent medical attention. We hardly had a few minutes to prepare.

The nurses on duty promptly arranged whatever was asked for – emergency trolley, intubation tray, two oxygen sources, suction apparatus and the Noccarc V310 ventilator, the latest addition to the ICU. There was a rush of activities as everyone took up their posts. We had a life to save!

The patient arrived, with monitors bearing grim stats.

The next few minutes were critical.

The crew jumped into action. Intubation and ventilation to ensure 100% oxygen saturation, a central line for emergency drugs and an arterial line to monitor the blood pressure and blood gas levels; everything was performed with professionalism and team support. Within half an hour the patient was ready for prone positioning, a recommended procedure to improve the lung oxygenation process, which also required high-level skills.

Such unpredictability being the norm, the efficiency of the tools at your disposal is as crucial as that of your team. So, it was gratifying to know that the new ventilator Noccarc V310 – mentored in our unit, and later received as a donation – had got our backs. That day, the V310 helped us save a life.

What ultimately matters in ICU management is efficient teamwork and preparedness along with reliable life-saving machines.

While skating on thin ice, safety is in speed!

Dr Prachee Sathe
MD FRCP FCCCM, Director ICU
Ruby Hall Clinic, Pune

It was with this vision, of standing by our health workers in times of extreme crisis, in mind that the IIT Kanpur Ventilator Consortium was formed on 29 March 2020. In the ninety days that followed, this task force would help a young robotics startup, Nocca Robotics, use its skills to build a ventilator in the face of the Covid-19 pandemic. Nocca had just created the initial (alpha) prototype of an 'invasive ventilator'. By late June, the first batch of the high-quality ventilators (Noccarc V310) was ready after three design iterations, safety testing, pre-clinical and clinical validation. A product development process that normally takes eighteen to twenty-four months was accelerated to three months, and the outcome was not just an 'acceptable' product, but a world-class one.

We were privileged to co-lead this task force of twenty people and get a ringside view of what the post-Covid world of business might look like. It was a crash course in navigating a world of dynamic and uncertain demand, volatile global sourcing, regulatory haziness and sceptical customers. It was also about life lessons centred around groups of people collaborating to create magic. Collaboration between the youth and the older generation, between top science and engineering institutions and business incubators, between a startup and an SME (small and medium-sized enterprise) and between individuals living across the world, working remotely and virtually, using Zoom and WhatsApp. In short, this is a story of collaborative social impact.

Even as we were working on the ventilator project, we had realized how priceless these lessons could be. Srikant's wife, Sudha, casually suggested one day that a book could be a good way of sharing these lessons with others. We jumped at the idea and that is how this book came to be.

We hope this true story that reveals how the limitations of time, resources and infrastructure can be catapults to success, inspires people to think about innovation and change. This is a story relevant to a new future with constant and accelerated changes, and new ways of working. At its heart, it's very much a story based in India and also one that has traversed the world.

The book has two broad sections. The first section, The Ninety-Day Saga, includes seventeen chapters that describe how the ventilator idea was conceived, the task force was assembled and brought into mission mode, and the product innovations envisaged to win over a sceptical medical fraternity while coping with regulatory uncertainty and a global lockdown. It also has stories that provide fascinating insights into what it takes to get things done in India, especially in manufacturing. The eight chapters in the second section, Big Hopes for the Future, are about dreaming audaciously in a rapidly changing world. They lay out an optimistic view that the pandemic has actually strengthened India's future trajectory, notwithstanding the GDP hiccups in 2020–21.

To say that Covid-19 has changed everyone's lives in 2020 would be an understatement. Undoubtedly, it did the same for both of us. But it has also made us very hopeful about our country and the world, for 2021 and beyond.

As we end this strange and unexpected year, we are filled with both the hope and confidence that Indians and India's institutions will emerge stronger from the pandemic and shape the reinvention of business in the post-Covid world.

Srikant Sastri and Amitabha Bandyopadhyay
December 2020

The Cast of Characters

Nocca Robotics

Nikhil Kurele and Harshit Rathore: the founders

Tushar Agarwal: the tech whiz

Asim Thakurta: the adult in the room

Project Leads

Srikant Sastri

Professor Amitabha Bandyopadhyay

Guru–Mentors

Saurabh Srivastava: serial entrepreneur angel and VC investor, institution builder (NASSCOM, TiE, Indian Angel Network, Indian Venture Capital Association), Padma Shri

Ajai Chowdhry: HCL founder, industry icon, Padma Bhushan

Medtech CEO Mentors

Sanjay Banerjee: highly well-connected, helpful, dependable

Sanjiv Verma: manufacturer at heart

Rakesh Bhargava: calmness personified, gets things done

Pavan Choudary: policy guru, Chanakya

Other Senior Mentors

Rajesh Raizada: there's no supply chain that he can't control

Arun Seth: industry veteran, the most well-networked person known to the project leads

Padmaja Ruparel: President at Indian Angel Network, Forbes 2018 W-Power Trailblazer, one of Fortune India's 'Most Powerful Women' of 2018

Deepak Saluja: sales expert

IIT Kanpur's Incubator (Startup Incubation and Innovation Centre) Team

Nikhil Agarwal: dynamic CEO, fundraiser with government relationships par excellence

Aditi Kumar: the dynamo who took the lead on everything to do with the product

Rahul Patel: synonymous with resourcefulness, mastered the supply chain

Others: Abhijit Sathe (manufacturing), Udayan Chandra (product training), Yogi Srivastava (financial and legal matters), Ravi Pandey (intellectual property law)

The Ventilator Project Timeline

Prime Minister's appeal

16 March	Prime Minister Narendra Modi launches the Covid-19 Solution Challenge through mygov.in
	The challenge is circulated among the portfolio companies of IIT Kanpur's incubator
21 March	Amitabha follows up with some of them, including Nocca Robotics

Six days before the task force is formed

23 March	IIT Kanpur's startup, Nocca Robotics, responds with interest to make ventilators
24 March	First meeting with four professors of IIT Kanpur, Dr Deepak Padmanabhan and a local manufacturer
25 March	Director of IIT Kanpur releases a video of Amitabha announcing IIT Kanpur's plan to make an ICU ventilator from scratch
26 March	Amitabha is introduced to The Bridge Ventilator Consortium
	Late-night call with Dr Govind Rajan of University of California, Irvine, USA
	Nocca's pressure-controlled ventilator concept is validated by Dr Rajan

27 March	Amitabha discusses ways of supporting the ventilator project with Srikant and Saurabh
	Srikant creates a WhatsApp group, names it 'India Overcomes COVID'
	Task force formation begins

The ninety-day saga

29 March	The first Zoom meeting of the task force takes place
5 April	Pressure-controlled ventilator prototype V110 is ready with simple mobile application
	Plans made for the next version, V210
9 April	Government of India steps in to help ship required components from Singapore
18 April	Manufacturing MOU is signed with AVI Healthcare
28 April	Manufacturing MOU is signed with PSU, Bharat Dynamics Ltd (BDL)
16 May	Ventilator V310 with both pressure and volume control modes and new user interface (UI) is ready
19 May	V310 successfully clears compliance test IEC 60601-1 in Pune
1 June	Endurance testing starts at Ruby Hall Clinic, Pune
5 June	Nocca signs manufacturing licence agreement with AVI Healthcare
8 June	Unexpected demo scheduled at Directorate General of Health Services (DGHS), but due to non-availability of oxygen cylinder, features are not demonstrated
15 June	The first five manufactured units are ready with Nocca Robotics in Pune
19 June	DGHS clears V310 with all specifications after the second demo

26 June	V310 successfully clears patient testing at Ruby Hall Clinic, Pune
	V310 is certified as fit to be used in the ICU

Four days before the task force is disbanded

29 June	V310 is tested and approved by two prestigious hospitals in Gurgaon – Medanta and Artemis
July 1	The last meeting of the task force

After the task force is disbanded

8 July	First meeting with the distributors
13 July	First commercial dispatch by AVI Healthcare to Neon Hospital, Dombivli, Maharashtra
15 July	First commercial dispatch by Nocca Robotics to Petronet LNG

A Ventilator Primer

The purpose of breathing is two-fold: (1) To absorb oxygen from the air and send it to our cells where it oxidizes (burns under controlled conditions) sugar to produce energy; and (2) to expel carbon dioxide (CO_2), the end product of this oxidation process so that the blood pH does not become acidic. Normally, it happens through an intricate, but apparently seamless, interplay of our brain, nervous system, muscles and lungs. The respiratory centre of the brain instructs the muscles, through several intermediaries, to contract which results in expansion of the chest cavity, thereby creating a negative air pressure that allows the lungs to suck in air. Within the lungs, there are small bubbles, called alveoli, where gas exchange takes place, and CO_2-rich air is readied for expulsion while oxygen-rich air defuses from the lungs to the blood stream, which carries the oxygen to all the cells of the body. During exhalation, the muscles relax, the chest cavity compresses and the CO_2-rich air is exhaled. Thus, we, and other mammals, breathe through the creation of a negative pressure environment around the lungs, while all amphibians with lungs, for example, frogs, breathe through the creation of positive pressure.

A person may suffer respiratory failure for a variety of reasons. Type I respiratory failure generally occurs due to suboptimal gas exchange. A number of underlying causes may give rise to such failure. For example, (1) a set of conditions that primarily originate at the interface between the lungs and the blood stream; or (2) pathologies leading to low-oxygen status in the body such as asthma which causes severe narrowing of the airways. One such condition is acute respiratory distress syndrome (ARDS) wherein fluid accumulates at the interface between the lungs and the blood stream, and thus oxygen cannot defuse into the blood stream. Type II respiratory failures happen due to compromised processes that do not allow the creation of the adequate negative pressure environment around the lungs, which may be due to neuronal or muscle problems that might have been caused by salt imbalance. Some disease conditions cause significant reduction of the surface area for gas exchange at the level of the airsacs, thus compromising the expulsion of CO_2 from blood.

A ventilator is a machine that helps a patient breathe if they cannot do it adequately on their own. However, ventilators act by creating a positive pressure environment around the lungs, which means air is forcibly pumped inside the chest cavity to force the alveoli to undergo gas exchange. This is known as mechanical ventilation.

The mechanical ventilation in its simplest form is manually pumping air into the patient's lung using an Ambu bag. In an Ambu bag, the rescuer manually compresses an inflatable bag causing the air to be force-fed into the patient's lungs. In an advanced form, the compression and relaxation of the Ambu bag can be controlled automatically which, in theory, can sustain ventilation for a long time. However, that is generally not the case as Ambu-bag-based ventilators cannot respond rapidly to the varying needs of injured, delicate lungs. In simple terms, as these devices operate through mechanical compression of a fixed-volume reservoir, there is always an inertia which cannot be rapidly altered based on the patient's need, while in most cases a respiratory device must respond to such rapidly changing needs. Thus, the Government of India did not prescribe the use of Ambu-bag-based ventilators on Covid-19 patients who often suffer from severe respiratory problems.

There are other types of mechanical ventilators such as transport ventilators and neonatal ventilators. The most sophisticated of the mechanical ventilators are the ICU ventilators.

ICU ventilators have a very sophisticated control of gas (air or a mixture of air and oxygen) delivery. These ventilators use pressure and flow sensors to accurately determine the volume, duration and pressure at which gas should be delivered to the patient. The use of these sensors allows these ventilators to rapidly adjust to the varying needs of the patient's inhalation/exhalation requirements.

The method of mechanical ventilation, including ventilation by ICU ventilators, can be broadly divided into two categories – non-invasive ventilation and invasive ventilation. Non-invasive ventilation, or NIV, differs from invasive ventilation in the interface between the ventilator and the patient. In NIV, the gas is pumped in and out of the patient's lungs via a face mask. Whereas in invasive ventilation, the gas is pumped in and out of the patient's lung using an invasive artificial tube, known as an endotracheal tube, which goes directly into the lungs via the mouth and windpipe.

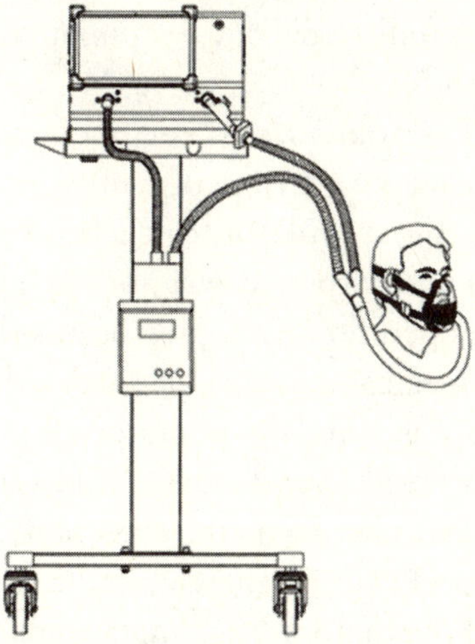

Non-Invasive Ventilation

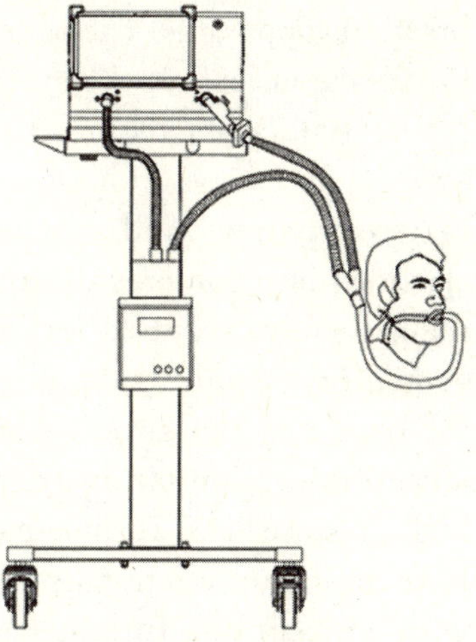

Invasive Ventilation

NIV has its own advantages. This mode of ventilation is used for patients suffering from mild to moderate respiratory distress. In such patients, sometimes the use of invasive ventilation can do more harm than good. Also, the NIV machine is more forgiving in terms of ventilation parameter settings, in case a senior intensivist or respiratory therapist is not available during an emergency. A basic form of the NIV can be found even at homes in the form of a CPAP or BiPAP machine, which is used to treat sleep apnea. However, the NIV mode of ventilation suffers from two problems: (1) there is leak of air at the interface of the mask and the skin around the mouth and on the nose, thus a sophisticated leak compensation process has to be built into the ICU ventilator to ensure that the desired volume of air is sent to the chest cavity; and (2) it also demands that the neuromuscular apparatus associated with breathing is fully functional and the patient is fully conscious. Often, a patient who is in a critical condition gets too fatigued from using this mode of ventilation or is incapable of overcoming severe respiratory failure. In such cases invasive ventilation is used. It provides better control over externally supported breaths as air is supplied straight into the chest cavity, bypassing the requirement of the rest of the breathing apparatus. The patient is fully rested due to minimized breathing, at least in the initial phase.

All ventilators require two gas sources, air and medical oxygen, for its operation. Apart from the interface of ventilation between patient and machine, the ventilator can also be classified into compressor-driven and turbine-driven, based on the gas source required for their operation. Compressor-based ventilators require compressed medical-grade air as a driver for operating the device. This air is generally compressed at a central location far away from the ICU and transported via high-pressure lines. Turbine-based ventilators, on the other hand, have an inbuilt electrically powered turbine and can make do with ambient air. Turbine-based ventilators offer much more independence and help bridge the gap between infrastructure supply and healthcare demand.

For both types of ventilators, medical oxygen has to be supplied either from an oxygen cylinder or the central oxygen supply system via a wall mount. From either of the sources, the oxygen can be supplied either at high pressure or low pressure using appropriate pneumatic fittings. The pressure of the oxygen depends on the mode of oxygen control in the ventilator. If the oxygen is electronically controlled, the ventilator is supplied with high-pressure oxygen, but if the oxygen is manually controlled using a flow meter, low-pressure oxygen is supplied to the ventilator. Depending on the condition of the patient, the percentage of oxygen in the air mixture (FiO_2) that is delivered to the patient may be varied. One way of varying FiO_2 is to control the oxygen flow through an external valve at the port where oxygen is being mixed with air. A more sophisticated way is to build FiO_2 into the ventilator so that it does not depend on any other function of the ventilator, for example, the flow rate.

An ICU ventilator should have the ability to deliver a set amount of volume (volume control mode) or at a set amount of pressure (pressure control mode). In the volume control mode, the ventilator will deliver the same volume during each ventilation cycle. The volume is measured automatically using flow sensors. However, depending on the condition of the lung, the pressure on it may be too high in volume control mode causing what is referred to as barotrauma. It should be noted that Ambu-bag-based ventilator design, if used on an ARDS patient, is particularly prone to causing barotrauma. In the pressure control mode, the clinician sets a pressure that the ventilator will deliver during each respiratory cycle. Again, depending on the condition of the lung, fixing the pressure may result in inadequate or excessive volume of air to be delivered, which can cause other physiological problems. The clinician makes the choice of the delivery mode depending on the patient's condition, and thus an ICU ventilator must be equipped with both of these delivery modes.

(This primer was authored in collaboration with Dr Prachee Sathe, ICU Director at Ruby Hall Clinic, Pune; Dr Deepak Padmanabhan, Assistant Professor, Sri Jayadeva Institute of Cardiovascular Sciences and Research, Bengaluru; and Tushar Agarwal, from Nocca Robotics.)

THE NINETY-DAY SAGA

1

The Phone Call that Started It All

On 16 March 2020, India had recorded sixty cases of Covid-19. The pandemic had only just begun to imprint itself on the national psyche. The World Health Organization had declared Covid-19 a global pandemic just five days prior, on 11 March, when the number of cases had reached 118,000 across 114 countries. Some optimistic forecasts predicted that Indians with their mighty immune systems that had been hardened by disease as well as their capacity for endurance thanks to scorching summers, would stop the virus in its tracks. As a precautionary measure, India had already banned incoming flights from the European Union, Turkey and the UK. Some states like Delhi had prohibited gatherings of more than fifty people. The government machinery had started to move on other fronts too.

When the Prime Minister of India announced a Covid-19 Solution Challenge on 16 March, nearly 500 kilometres away in Kanpur, Professor Amitabha Bandyopadhyay sent out news of the challenge as an SOS to all IIT Kanpur-incubated startups, hoping a few would have the products or services necessary to fight the pandemic. Several came forth with solutions ranging from hand sanitizers, PPEs, N95 face masks, diagnostic kits and portable respirators.

Then came the pitch for a ventilator by a robotics venture named Nocca Robotics. There was a simplicity and elegance to the proposal for building a high-quality life-saving device that immediately caught Amitabha's attention. Until then, Nocca Robotics had been in the business of making robots to clean solar panels without using water.

Nocca Robotics was the brainchild of Nikhil Kurele and Harshit Rathore, both 2016 graduates of IIT Kanpur (IIT-K). Nikhil had grown up in Shahdol, a small town in Madhya Pradesh, and was a 'badmaash' at school. Academics was not a priority for him. Although he fell in love with maths in class eight, he remained terrible at other subjects. In the class ten board exams, when he got 96% in maths but only 71% overall, Nikhil's parents packed him off to Kota for his final two school years so he wouldn't be able to keep up his 'errant' ways. It was in Kota that he prepared for his IIT entrance exam.

Soon Nikhil was in IIT-K, where he developed an interest in robotics and became the secretary of the Robotics Club. A summer internship at the Frugal Innovation in Design and Technology Centre at IIT-K, followed by a second one as a design engineer at Tata Technologies, honed his interest in design. A ten-month stint at Bajaj Auto after graduating from IIT-K gave him the exposure to automation in assembly and machining processes. And with these pieces in place, the path to creating Nocca Robotics had been paved, especially once he met Harshit Rathore.

Although Harshit, a local from Kanpur, was a chemistry student at IIT-K, his heart was in motorsport. He was the technical lead for the Baja SAE All-Terrain Vehicle project on campus. A summer internship at Tata Motors and ten months in fabricated metal products manufacturing completed his transition from chemistry to robotics. Harshit and Nikhil shared a love for SAE motorsport and racing at 140–150 kmph on the IIT Kanpur airstrip was one of the ways in which they bonded. They would import components to build cars, using the money sent by their parents meant for tuition fees and wait for the club to reimburse it. Besides a love for motorsport, the duo also shares the same date of birth (though, as is common in India, Nikhil's official date of birth is different).

Nocca Robotics finally lifted off in April 2017 at the Startup Incubation and Innovation Centre (SIIC), IIT-K's incubation centre. Despite the usual startup hiccups of product development, initial customer adoption, cash flows and mentoring, they obtained seed funding from SIIC and Villgro and mentoring from several IIT-K alumni. Their big break came with initial orders from Adani Power and Mahindra Susten, and early conversations with Renew, Tata Voltas and Azure Power. This provided them with confidence which was bolstered by a series of funds raised from the Indian Angel Network (IAN) Fund in June 2019. With orders in hand, and now money in the bank too, Nocca Robotics was all set to build their business.

But on 21 March, the call from Amitabha changed the startup's course completely.

Nikhil had first responded to the call by offering to only assemble ventilators, then made a pitch to design a new one. By that time, India had recorded only 471 cases and 8 deaths, but the government had already begun preparing the country for social distancing by implementing a voluntary 'janata curfew' from 7 a.m. to 9 p.m. on the previous day. By 24 March, Amitabha was convinced, along with the IIT-K Director Professor Abhay Karandikar, that the campus incubator would need to work with Nocca to build a new ventilator from scratch.

The very same day, Amitabha brainstormed with a small group of Mechanical Engineering professors (Sameer Khandekar, Arun Saha and J Ramkumar) and Dr Deepak Padmanabhan, a cardiologist from Bangalore who is one of the clinical mentors of the incubator. Various ventilator designs were deliberated upon including an Ambu-bag-based design. Ambu-bags are handheld devices used to help patients breathe especially in out-of-hospital situations. However, Dr Padmanabhan was very clear that only a full-fledged ICU ventilator would serve the purpose of saving Covid-19 patients. This was clearly a daunting challenge considering that Nikhil and Harshit had never seen a functioning ICU ventilator, let alone designed one.

However, they decided to take up the challenge.

There were many factors behind their decision, the first of which was of course, purely emotional – they wanted to serve the nation in its hour of crisis. IIT training develops in students not just the confidence to tackle any challenge but also an affinity towards being challenged. The crazier it is, the more they love it. There were two practical considerations as well. They realized that working on the ventilator project would allow them to operate their factory during the lockdown. And since such an important project was very likely to be generously funded, they would be able to hold onto their engineering team at Nocca Robotics. With this belief, they gave their hundred percent commitment to the project.

On 25 March, the director of IIT Kanpur, and a huge champion of the project, Professor Abhay Karandikar, posted on all his social media handles about this ambitious project. This gave the project much needed visibility, which brought in offers of collaboration and help kept pouring in. On 26 March, Amitabha received an email from Professor Ashutosh Sharma, Secretary at the Department of Science of Technology, Government of India, who is also an alumnus of IIT-K and a member of its faculty on lien to Government of India. Professor Sharma introduced Amitabha to a global team of volunteers – The Bridge Ventilator Consortium – who were helping teams from different countries to develop ventilators. One of the members of the team was Dr Govind Rajan, Clinical Professor, Department of Anesthesiology and Perioperative Care at the University of California in Irvine. Amitabha set up a meeting between the Nocca Robotics team and Dr Govind Rajan at 11 p.m. IST on 26 March 2020. Dr Rajan began by explaining how an Ambu-bag-based ventilator works and how to design it quickly. After he finished, the Nocca team politely informed him that their clinical mentor had urged them to only pursue an ICU ventilator and nothing else. Dr Rajan agreed with the advice given but was sceptical if this could be pulled off given all the constraints and the high-level precision needed. Like a magician pulling a rabbit out of a hat, Nikhil suddenly showed everyone a prototype of an ICU ventilator, and even Amitabha was stunned.

Nikhil and Harshit explained quite nonchalantly how they had got this done in the last three days by working almost non-stop. Two other IIT-K alumni were stuck in Nikhil and Harshit's Pune apartment during the sudden lockdown in Maharashtra – their batchmate Abhishek Kulkarni and their junior Tushar Agarwal. Soon after the 24 March meeting with the director, the four of them had divided up work among themselves to read about different aspects of the ventilator.

Harshit and Tushar focused on the electronic circuits of an ICU ventilator and quickly created one mostly by using the parts used in their solar panel cleaning robots. Nikhil and Abhishek read up about the mechanical aspects and design to make the CAD (computer-aided design) model of their first prototype. They consulted several YouTube videos and learnt what mechanical components would be needed to create a ventilator prototype. With brilliant improvisation and a little luck on their side, they found a hobby store in Pune that stocked several robotics components. They began working on the prototype.

Ventilators need air pumps; for the prototype, they used a pump used in fish tanks. They needed pressure sensors. From the store, they bought pressure sensors meant for use in hobby drones (unmanned aerial vehicles). By the evening of 25 March, they had the prototype working. Abhishek Kulkarni, who had some experience in designing apps, developed one for the ventilator by the next evening, just in time for the demo for Dr Rajan.

Dr Rajan asked some probing questions about the design and about contingency measures to source components during the impending global lockdown. When Harshit and Nikhil defended their design with confidence, and explained their sourcing plans, he exclaimed, 'I wish they were in the US working with our teams here!'

Amitabha walked away from the meeting confident that the Nocca team had passed its first big test. The next morning, he called Srikant and veteran serial entrepreneur Saurabh Srivastava to brief them about the meeting with Dr Rajan. His newfound confidence rubbed off on both of them; they all agreed that the IIT-K ventilator project should be a top priority, and that a task force should be created.

As the first step, a WhatsApp group was created on 27 March – 'India Overcomes COVID'. The stage was now set.

On this date, India's Covid-19 toll had risen to 871 cases and 21 deaths.

KEY TAKEAWAYS

The power of belief is hard to match.

- Unexpected big opportunities often appear out of nowhere.
- The fear of the unknown may initially be discouraging.
- Personal confidence and great teamwork help drive this fear away.
- A higher purpose – a national or global cause – creates unmatched strong beliefs.

2

Assembling the Star Cast

India went into lockdown on 25 March 2020, just as Covid-19 cases had begun to rise in the country. The IIT-K ventilator needed to be available in record time if it was to fight this pandemic. Though the prototype had passed the first test with Dr Govind Rajan on 26 March, we realized conventional ways of organizing ourselves and building a product would not work at such an exceptional time. Instead, we needed a wide variety of expertise: from medical technology producers, doctors and biomedical engineers to manufacturing experts and savvy entrepreneurs. Together with Saurabh Srivastava, on 27 March 2020, we drew up a wish list for our task force, the most important criteria being people with their hearts in the right place, and who could contribute their time and energy during a pandemic.

The first person we called was Sanjay Banerjee, Srikant's batchmate from IIT Kanpur as well as the Indian Institute of Management Calcutta (IIM-C). They had known each other for over forty years, and Sanjay had decades of pharma and medical tech experience in various companies. He was also the first port of call every time Srikant had a medical emergency.

At IIM-C, Sanjay was nicknamed Reuter, because of his widespread access to information and his wide networks and connections. True to form, he consulted Dr Prakash Keshaviah and Yashdeep Kumar almost immediately for an expert review of the alpha prototype. The director of dialysis at the Himalayan Institute Hospital Trust, Dr Keshaviah came with a strong background in biomedical engineering, while Yashdeep, a medtech rockstar, brought with him twenty-four years of experience at Stryker Corporation, and is presently the Vice President of Global Innovation. Very few people know the global medical technology scene as well as he does. We would reach out to both Dr Keshaviah and Yashdeep on a couple of more occasions for their feedback. So, as the initial assessment of the prototype got underway, Sanjay began working on the supply chain and manufacturing end of the project to identify the right mentors for the task force.

Pavan Choudary got the next call. Srikant had met him in 1990 when Pavan had interviewed for a job at Tara Sinha–McCann Erickson, the advertising agency Srikant was working for at the time. Over the years, Pavan and Srikant had stayed in touch, owing in large part to the former's amazing people skills. On his LinkedIn page, a recommendation reads, 'I admire his capacity to always find time for his friends and balance his professional life with his philanthropic pursuits and varied interests from writing to conducting sessions for the senior bureaucrats, politicians and CEOs from the industry.' As the India CEO of Vygon (a French medical devices company) for twenty-two years and now chairman of the Medical Technology Association of India, he has been at the forefront of industry initiatives. What we wanted was his perspective on policy and regulatory frameworks and the competition.

Next, Saurabh turned his focus to a very important candidate, Ajai Chowdhry, founder of HCL Technologies. He asked him whether he would be willing to come on board. We wanted his experience of running India's most aggressive sales company and largest manufacturing business. Ajai, in turn, invited his former HCL supply chain colleague Rajesh Raizada. As soon as

Rajesh agreed, Ajai sent us a message: 'Please send him the Bill of Materials so he can get started. His mind is already buzzing with ideas!'

This mentor group was completed with the addition of the dynamic Padmaja Ruparel, President of the Indian Angel Network (IAN) and a managing partner at IAN Fund.

The fellowship of the eight mentors was now ready to turn the ventilator project into reality. But we needed to ensure that the Nocca founders would not be deluged with advice. So, we came up with a 'three pillar' structure almost intuitively, with the Nocca founders as the left pillar, the mentors being the right and the IIT-K incubator team at the centre. Seven members from the incubator team – Nikhil Agarwal, Aditi Kumar, Rahul Patel, Abhijit Sathe, Udayan Chandra, Yogi Srivastava and Ravi Pandey – were assigned to the task force to connect Nócca with the mentors.

The task force also brought in two doctors to periodically weigh in with their thoughts. The first was Dr Deepak Padmanabhan, who is a member of the medtech panel at IIT-K that reviews innovations, besides being on committees that reviewed the Government of India's Biotechnology Industry Research Assistance Council (BIRAC) – an autonomous entity under the Department of Biotechnology, grants. He had a bird's-eye view of the medtech innovation landscape in India and had returned to the country after a stint at Mayo Clinic in the US. He worked at the Narayana Institute of Cardiac Sciences, Bangalore, and is currently an assistant professor at Sri Jayadeva Institute of Cardiovascular Sciences and Research. One other doctor – Dr Dileep Raman, a pulmonary and critical care specialist and co-founder of Bangalore-based tele-ICU startup Cloudphysician – was also brought in. For occasional advice on policy matters, Amitabha identified Rahul Raj, an engineer from the Indian Institute of Technology (BHU) Varanasi, whose current passion is to develop energy storage products.

The task force was now ready: eight mentors; six members from the IIT-K incubator; the two Nocca founders; and the talented Tushar Agarwal who had recently joined the Nocca team. An excellent group of doctors acted as our sounding board. We now needed to get cracking and deliver results in a record time frame.

Often, assembling a star cast is easier than getting them to work together. The results are harder to predict when people do not know each other too well. In a popular TED Talk[1], Harvard Business School Professor Amy Edmondson describes 'teaming', whereby people come together quickly (and often temporarily) to solve new, urgent or unusual problems, and talks about how hundreds of unrelated individuals came together during the incredible rescue of thirty-three miners trapped half a mile underground in Chile in 2010. On the other hand, where the Indian Premier League (IPL) is concerned, a diverse group of players come together for six to seven weeks every year, and while some teams do well, others play well below their potential year after year. The first few people, who form the core nucleus, determine the success of a team. This core must strongly believe in the mission, bring a skill unique to each member, and come in with resilience, a learning mindset and a sense of humour.

For our task force, we wanted to ensure all our members could come together to form a cohesive unit. As four more members joined – Arun Seth, former chairman of British Telecom India and an ace problem solver; Rakesh Bhargava, a medtech veteran with an experience of twenty-two years at the German company Fresenius Kabi; Sanjiv Verma, former Managing Director of Baxter India, armed with manufacturing expertise; and Deepak Saluja, medtech sales expert – we were now ready to take off.

Sunday, 29 March was set as the date when this star cast would meet for the first time.

KEY TAKEAWAYS

Assembling a star team takes much more than simply bringing together a team of stars.

- The first few people are crucial. Their presence will act like a magnet, and they will form the core of the team.
- Others will join a mission if they can see a meaningful purpose in it. The best way to find such people is by first tapping into the core team's networks. A more cohesive team can be built through referrals.
- Finding high-quality, action-oriented individuals with relevant expertise, people skills, resilience and a sense of humour is the key to success.

STARTER KIT

STEP 1: The purpose of a task force should be clearly defined. Is it about fighting a pandemic or a natural disaster? Or is it an idea that can lead to India's equivalent of an Amazon or a Google and can change the world while making money?

STEP 2: List the skill sets required to make the task force extraordinary. Expertise is important, but more so is ensuring that the team members are resilient doers with good people skills.

STEP 3: Think of the first three people in your own network who can meet your criteria. These individuals should be excited by the core purpose of your project and not have conflicting goals. Talk to them, and pitch your idea with conviction. Once you have found the first three members, tap into their networks to bring in others with a similar vision and experience.

Notes

1. Edmondson, Amy. October 2017. 'How to Turn a Group of Strangers into a Team.' TED video, 12:59. https://www.ted.com/talks/amy_edmondson_how_to_turn_a_group_of_strangers_into_a_team#t-2185

3

The Daily Zoom Call

When the task force came together for the first time on 29 March, the number of global Covid-19 cases had crossed 660,000. India had recorded 1,091 cases at the time and was just getting used to the lockdown announced by Prime Minister Narendra Modi. The entire nation looked ahead with determination mixed with a fear of the unknown. What would happen next?

It was a Sunday, so the task force decided that we would all meet over Zoom at noon. Little did we know at the time that this video conference would come to dominate our lives for the next ninety days. The meeting became a clarion call for us, a glue that would hold us together, backed by regular WhatsApp exchanges as a second layer of adhesive. We had also created smaller and more focused groups for the areas of Product, Sourcing, Manufacturing, Corporate Social Responsibility, Regulatory Compliance and Training.

Each group now grew animated, and the action continued through the night. The younger members, mostly the Nocca founders and the IIT-K incubator team, would go to sleep at 5 a.m., just as older members like the authors would be waking up. We were literally following the sun, the moon and the stars!

On most days, as discussions would stretch well into the afternoon, some members would discreetly turn off their videos and start with their lunch. But the clanging of utensils gave their game away. As weeks passed, we saw how the locked-down members' hairstyles and clothes evolved and spent the first five minutes of the call exchanging jokes about intriguing new haircuts received from spouses or kids!

Somewhere in mid-April, the Ministry of Home Affairs issued a security advisory that Zoom meetings may not be secure and could be hacked easily by miscreants. For a moment this made us a little worried. However, everyone grew comfortable when Zoom issued its product updates and the use of passwords became commonplace.

Our meetings would first focus on updates regarding product development, supply chain management, manufacturing partnerships, regulatory issues and funding. Then we would brainstorm about areas that needed more discussion. Invariably, the updates and brainstorming sessions would mesh into one another. Given the lack of a formal hierarchy or organizational structure that could bring discipline to such meetings, it fell upon us to steer the conversation back on track. In the first meeting itself, it was decided that the Nocca team's time would be best spent focusing on product development, while other task force members would take the lead on areas like managing the supply chain, arranging permits and permissions for travel and shipments, raising funds and augmenting the Nocca team's progress with inputs from the team members.

Typically, each idea or initiative would be pursued by a specialist group comprising one Nocca founder, a few mentors from the task force and someone from the IIT-K incubator. The external mentor provided experience-based guidance, the founders did the tech work, while the incubator did the rest of the heavy lifting. The task force had accidentally stumbled upon a structure that worked well for operations in mission mode.

The Nocca founders knew the mentors had committed time to the task force, so they took the noon call seriously, often treating it like an exam where they'd be asked probing questions.

The calls became a daily, almost sacrosanct ninety-minute ritual, and it felt sacrilegious to miss one. This noon-time routine continued uninterrupted through ninety days, except for one time, on a Saturday, when the call was rescheduled to 5.30 p.m. to accommodate a member based in the US. Every day the task force would solve new challenges, take up even more ambitious targets and would be greeted with exhilarating tech updates from Tushar on behalf of the Nocca team. We all looked forward to it. Notwithstanding the age difference, everyone behaved like wide-eyed kids during these meetings.

The working mechanism was now in place, and the task force had set up an ambitious agenda for itself. The first on the 'to do' list was to quickly finalize a ventilator design that would be a useful and efficient aid to Covid-19 patients in the ICU. And at the same time, be easy to manufacture – considering the choke of the global supply chain due to the world-wide lockdown – while being totally safe and reliable.

KEY TAKEAWAYS

Remote collaboration tools are transforming work habits positively.

- A fixed routine of meetings goes a long way in making it into a habit.
- Lay out a formal or semi-formal agenda for each meeting to keep discussions focused.
- A combination of videoconferencing, messaging, phone and email platforms ensures round-the-clock progress.

STARTER KIT

STEP 1: Use the calendar effectively to pick the days and hours that work for most members, especially the key players. Others may need to make a few adjustments. Block everyone's calendar for the lifespan of the task force. Resist the temptation to periodically change schedules to accommodate someone. Accept that not everyone can attend every meeting. For less intense projects during non-crisis periods, weekly calls should suffice, if supported by more frequent meetings of sub-groups.

STEP 2: Based on the comfort of most members, pick a videoconferencing platform and a messaging platform. The meeting title (on the videoconferencing platform) and names of WhatsApp groups should reflect the ambition and purpose of the groups. Choose the technology that suits everyone.

STEP 3: Use both 'full quorum' and 'specialized forums' to build momentum. Everyone in the task force must meet regularly over video call to review and discuss common and bigger issues. Individual workstreams (for example, product development, regulatory approvals, funding) need more focused discussions within smaller groups. Use smaller WhatsApp groups and periodic video conferences as specialized forums for these aspects.

4

How Did They Design It So Fast?

Every IIT has some exceptionally bright students – even by IIT standards – who seem to score high grades without ever breaking a sweat. They are the ones who lend class notes to others or help solve difficult assignment problems when no one else can. Tushar Agarwal had been one such student during his college days. He had a cumulative points index (CPI) of 9.4 (out of 10) during his MTech at IIT-K. CPI is similar to the 'grade point average' at many universities. With interests spanning automobiles, robotics and Internet of Things (IoT), Tushar was also one of the coolest guys around. He had a 500cc methanol-fuelled motorcycle (developed at IIT-K's Engine Research Laboratory) and an Autonomous Navigation Vehicle (funded by The Boeing Company) under his belt.

When it came to designing a complicated machine like a ventilator in record time, Nikhil and Harshit knew that Tushar would be their saviour. '*Kyunki Tushar ki CPI high thi, isliyay isko yeh kaam diya* (We gave Tushar this job because his CPI was so high),' revealed Nikhil when Amitabha wondered in the early days who could understand the workings of an ICU ventilator by reading up and studying all the available material on this topic.

Thus began the journey. Nikhil and Harshit were confident that if Tushar told them what exactly to make, they could make it well. Tushar immersed himself into learning about the functioning of lungs and reading all that was there to read about the functioning of ICU ventilators. Medical textbooks, clinical literature, ventilator brochures of leading manufacturers – he read them all. While he did that, Nikhil took charge of the mechanical assembly as Harshit looked after the electronic controls. These were their respective areas of expertise from their IIT days when, as part of their Society of Automotive Engineers club activity, they had built a car for an international competition. Those skills were further tested and perfected when they started their business of manufacturing robots that could clean solar panels. The job of telling them what to do rested with Tushar, who had joined the Nocca team less than a month ago.

Their only missing area of expertise was software. The ventilator needed an app that would act as the interface to enable the electronic systems to run the mechanical systems. Nikhil and Harshit turned to Abhishek Kulkarni, their batchmate, who had developed an app for the 26 March meeting with Dr Govind Rajan. They knew Abhishek would be stranded in Pune for quite some time because of the lockdown. With Abhishek by their side, they developed the first version of the app. Elle Atma Vidya Prakash aka Khan (hostel nickname), another classmate of Nikhil and Harshit's, helped out with the electronics and firmware (software that is etched into the hardware) development.

The team smartly continued to follow the motto that had worked for them so well when they had developed their first prototype within seventy-two hours – use locally and easily available components whenever possible. To achieve this, they needed to understand the functioning of every component of a high-end ventilator very well so that they could substitute one component with an alternative without compromising the functionality of the ventilator.

Technical inputs started to pour in from the two clinical mentors – Dr Deepak Padmanabhan and Dr Dileep Raman. A third clinical mentor, Dr Prachee Sathe, had also come on board recently. Tushar would understand from them the requirements in terms of the inner workings of the machine and would convey it all to the rest of the Nocca Robotics team. Each midnight there would be a team meeting with Nikhil, Harshit, Tushar and Abhishek where ideas were debated. Decisions were taken and action plans finalized only when all four of them were in complete agreement. Harshit recalls how these brainstorming sessions would sometimes get really heated when the proponent of any idea would try and convince the other three who were just as incredibly gifted engineers. These intense brainstorming sessions ensured that they seldom barked up the wrong tree and got things right the first time, while ensuring that the speed of development was extraordinary.

For Tushar to meet his other 'goal' of presenting a new product feature or concept to the task force every three days, close interaction with the clinicians, among other things, was required. The team had unrestricted access to Dr Sathe and her team of doctors at Ruby Hall Clinic, Pune. The clinicians permitted Tushar to study their ventilators to understand the flow of air, and the control of the flow through an artificial lung. This allowed Tushar to fully grasp the theoretical concepts that he read in the literature and gave him ideas on how to implement the same. He would take those ideas to the brainstorming sessions where they would be perfected by his three other collegemates.

There were two additional critical factors that aided the speed of development. Pune is a hub of India's automobile industry and is home to many top-class companies with expertise in producing high-quality electronics and mechanical parts as well as structural components. One of Pune's celebrated industrialists, Mr Sudhir Mehta, the Chairman and Managing Director of

Pinnacle Industries, is a leading maker of automotive seats and interiors. He took the Nocca team under his wing, providing them preferential treatment at many of the fabrication shops in Pune to get their components readied at rapid speed. Task force member and one of the medtech mentors, Rakesh Bhargava, being based in Pune also helped open many other doors.

The other factor was cashflow. Nikhil Kurele tells us that Nocca Robotics' monthly expenses had always been modest in the past, and it was a new experience for him to see so much cash being used towards ventilator development. However, he did not have to worry about this problem. He and the team could happily focus on their midnight brainstorming sessions with the sole intent of narrowing down those practical technical solutions knowing full well that others in the task force would arrange the money.

However, in mid-May, the development hit a bad patch for the want of a good app. The app that Abhishek had earlier developed was never meant to be the final version. It was only a stopgap measure to help them test the machine and its features. Nocca paid a hefty sum to a third-party vendor for developing the final app which had many bugs that the vendor could not rectify in time. The desperate Nocca team and members of the task force approached big Indian corporates who have such core expertise. Many simply stated that it was beyond their capability to develop such an app, while a couple offered to do it but asked for one month. Nocca did not have that kind of time.

Once again, a young team of IIT-K alumni – Kshitij Jaggi, Kumar Shivang and Rishabh Sahu – co-founders of UrbanYogi, a startup with expertise in app development, came to the rescue. They developed the app in just seven days.

The ventilator design eventually went through three iterations (V110, V210 and finally V310) in response to the changing requirements of the Ministry of Health and Family Welfare, before the final version – the V310 – was approved and readied in just ninety days. It was a record by all standards. But at every stage, it was the sheer brilliance of this young team, superb planning, hard work and great camaraderie that made it possible to design this essential, complicated machine in a matter of months.

Through these ninety days, the product design heroes had to deal with a powerful, almost-villainous force, the uncertain and unknown availability of vital imported components. The heroes would be ready with their firmware and waiting for components to arrive while the formidable Rajesh Raizada and the tireless Rahul Patel fought hard to source them globally.

These battles, sometimes resembling scenes from a Kollywood or Bollywood thriller, were to provide heartbreaks and highs in the weeks to come.

KEY TAKEAWAYS

Bright inventors filled with idealism and a can-do spirit can create wonders.

- India's engineering colleges are full of bright, young people who have the ideas and skills to create great products.
- These young inventors want to build these world-class products well and without cutting corners.
- They also know how to face constraints and overcome them.

STARTER KIT (FOR YOUNG INVENTORS)

STEP 1: Pick some real problems to solve using your technology skills. India has a bagful of problems waiting to be solved in areas like agriculture, environment, waste management, urban planning, affordable housing, education, livelihoods, and more. The list is endless. Technology now provides India an opportunity to leapfrog conventional solutions and actually find radical answers.

STEP 2: Discard slow, traditional methods of building your product and your business. India needs solutions fast. Make plans to solve problems in an accelerated manner by bringing together the best technology team you can assemble. Young teams with the right motivation and energy can create magic.

STEP 3: Reach out to good incubators and ask them to help by finding the right mentors for yourself. Not just one mentor, but a team of mentors with complementary skills who can put you on a fast track by working with you to overcome bottlenecks.

5

Global Sourcing à la Rajinikanth

Rajesh Raizada is a product of the legendary PC wars of India in the 1990s, when domestic brands were slogging it out amongst themselves for market leadership. HCL was the market leader at the time but was constantly irritated by the 'upstart' Pertech Computers Ltd (PCL), now a defunct company. The competition relied on features and pricing and full-page newspaper ads were par for the course.

At the time Rajesh was still a newbie at HCL. One day in September 1996, he was summoned for an urgent meeting at HCL boss Shiv Nadar's residence. Rajesh was the youngest in the room. The war room was discussing ways to counter PCL's announcement of a PC priced at ₹24,999, which was yet to launch in the market. HCL wanted to get there quicker; they wanted to launch PCs at the impossible price of ₹19,999 by 17 October, in just two weeks. All Shiv Nadar and then HCL CEO Ajai Chowdhry said was, 'You guys figure out how to get this done.'

This moment became Rajesh's trial by fire in the 'sourcing' world. Over the next few days, PC486 motherboards and memory cards were flown in from HCL America, power supply units brought on the Rajdhani Express from Chennai, and monitors were sourced from local suppliers. All materials arrived by 12 October. The assembly began the next day, and the first

250 PCs were on the shelf by the 16 October. The deadline had been beaten with half a day to spare! Not even an action sequence in a Rajinikanth movie could be as exciting!

Within the next six months, Rajesh set up a supply chain for a monthly capacity of 20,000 PCs with the help of Tapesh Sinha, an influential member of the 1900-strong Indian community in Taiwan. Tapesh had long-standing relationships with Taiwanese companies that could supply to HCL. Acctel, his company, ended up becoming a partner for Rajesh and HCL for the next twenty-five years, helping to drive their entire sourcing strategy. In the price-sensitive PC business, where money can only be made through efficient sourcing, Tapesh became a great asset for HCL.

Rajesh no longer works with HCL, but when he joined the task force, the wheel came full circle. Rajesh once again turned to Tapesh for advice when faced with roadblocks on the issue of sourcing.

Between April and June 2020, every company was grappling with the challenge of sourcing raw materials and components, both because of the pandemic and due to some countries having moved away from doing business with China. Companies were looking for smarter ways to secure their sourcing. In the short term, thanks to Rajesh's guidance, the task force navigated through sourcing in a volatile global environment while trying to decide whether future profitability lay in smarter sourcing or through value addition beyond sourcing. The team balanced the need for best components with pricing, availability and the ability to ship to India. Agility, resourcefulness and support from a surprising quarter ensured that the sourcing process was not compromised.

When Rajesh joined the task force at the end of March, most aspects of the project were hazy and tentative: the ventilator design, product specifications and most certainly the one document that is gospel for sourcing experts – the bill of materials (BOM). The BOM is a list of raw materials, sub-assemblies, intermediate assemblies, sub-components, parts, and the quantities of each needed to manufacture the product. A sourcing expert would be lost without this. But because we needed to get a prototype ready by 15 May for approval by the Directorate General of Health Services (DGHS), the sourcing group was tasked with initiating the sourcing without the BOM. The BOM was not finalized until 19 June when the product design was accepted by DGHS and the task force.

A forty-five-day deadline, but no BOM! The sourcers now had to juggle with one eye on the deadline and the other on the BOM, which was more akin to working with a moving target, because product specifications were constantly changing as fresh inputs came in from experts and amendments were repeatedly announced in the government tender requirements. For instance, when the product design suddenly required flow sensors, this meant a change in three other components of the ventilator. The sourcing team was learning and improvising on the job to solve the challenges that came their way – further compounded by the global shortage in supply of components and the inability to ship them internationally or even domestically.

The sourcing team had two simple rules for scarce components with volatile availability: 'Grab what you can get' and 'Get samples from them all'. Luck played a role too. One supplier's website had mistakenly listed pressure sensors under the wrong category. Others missed it, but our team spotted it and immediately placed an order.

Printed circuit boards (PCBs) are important to all electronic gadgets because these thin boards connect different electronic components and provide mechanical support. The Nocca team had developed its first-level PCB design by 12 April and needed a manufacturer who could make this for us. With India under lockdown at the time, we looked for companies in Taiwan and China. We had almost finalized the deal with a Taiwanese company when a company in Pune reached out and agreed to our terms. Though their timelines were vague, we trusted them, and they delivered on time.

Our noon calls would often begin with a dose of dark lockdown humour that arose from sourcing challenges. For example, once we had placed an order for Honeywell flow sensors with their distributor in Chennai, and also paid a ₹1 lakh advance that Honeywell had insisted upon. But the sensors never arrived because the distributor had locked up his office and warehouse and gone away to his hometown in the interiors of Tamil Nadu. Frantic phone calls were made to no avail. There were also times when some key suppliers would suddenly go out of action because their factories had been placed in the 'Red Zone' – areas categorized by the government as having a large number of Covid-19 cases – and hence, they needed stricter containment guidelines. Once these areas were sealed off by the civic authorities, no movement was allowed in or out of the area.

Sometimes, these heartbreaks would lead to high-speed coordination involving several members of the task force. A consignment of power supply units and oxygen sensors was due to be transported from Ahmedabad to Pune by road. The distributor in Ahmedabad had his stock ready. But as luck would have it, the Ahmedabad police apparently discovered a quantity of drugs hidden inside PPE kits just the previous day. Heads rolled in the Ahmedabad administration, and no one could help us. Finally, a senior ex-bureaucrat advised our logistics partner to apply for permission to the Taluka headquarters. They got an approval and brought the consignment to Mumbai, where a Tata Ace was arranged, and the Mumbai Police was requested to allow them safe transit up to Pune.

When the sourcing team looks back now, of course they feel they could have done many things differently or even better. But, as Rajesh says, 'This was excellent work done amidst the highest level of ambiguity.'

The global lockdown triggered a debate, not just within the task force but also in government circles, about the levels of indigenization in ventilators and similar medical equipment. Out of the eighty-five V310 components, thirteen were sourced from outside India and accounted for 65% of the BOM value. The components – oxygen and flow and pressure sensors, power supply units, display screens, pump units and dehumidifiers – were partly sourced from Europe and the US, and partly from China, Taiwan or South East Asia. During the pandemic, inbound logistics had slowed down, while rising global demand increased the waiting period. The Sino-Indian border crisis of June 2020 brought additional challenges. As a result, local suppliers did not succeed in designing and producing power supply units and pumps.

Our experience tells us that 100% indigenization of input components is unlikely for several more years. India will find it hard to make semiconductors, sensors and certain power supply components locally. But should our target be 100% indigenization of input components at all, or should the focus be on adding more value in India during the product design and manufacturing process instead? For instance, Nocca imports components worth about ₹50,000, but the final product is a lot more valuable because of superior design, local components, software, manufacturing process, quality control and customer service. This allows Nocca to sell the ventilator in India at a price of ₹3 lakh or more. The bulk of the profits are retained in India by Nocca and other Indian suppliers, distributors, dealers, training partners and customer service partners.

Further, should this be India's national policy too? Instead of trying to compete with other countries in manufacturing low-value components, we can compete in the higher value-added ventilators market even if many of the components are imported. Expert advisor Yashdeep Kumar has similar views.

'Value creation is not in BOM or product cost. It is in sales, marketing and customer education.'[1] Multinational medical equipment suppliers have mastered this. Our sourcing team estimates that the Draeger ventilators imported from Germany are unlikely to have a BOM value of more than ₹1–1.5 lakh, but they sell for ₹10 lakh in the market. They charge for their brand, their expertise in integration, and everything else that Yashdeep has mentioned.

How do we deal with the issue of countries trying to move away from China and its impact on sourcing? The task force's sourcing team believed that if costs were important, China would be the viable choice, but if quality was important, we should buy the components from elsewhere. And if in the future a ban on Chinese imports is levied, we could shift to Taiwanese suppliers, even though the prices will be slightly higher. Moreover, the Nocca team was sceptical of the reliability of Chinese components. Initially, when the team had run a Chinese pump continuously for forty-five days, they were relieved when no problems emerged. But in subsequent batches of products from the same company, they got shoddy products.

Tapesh Sinha believes the shift away from China will not happen overnight but he recommends making a start quickly by building smart relationships with high-quality goods suppliers, 'Even if the volumes are small, work with the business development team of the company whose component is going to be used. Most manufacturers don't just want to sell, but also want their components incorporated in a strategic product that has long-term potential.'[2]

The trust that German, Swiss, Japanese or American medical device manufacturers have earned is, in part, due to their investment in good sourcing partners and the ability to engage these partners well. Rajesh wanted Nocca to do exactly this, invest in one or two smart professionals in the supply chain, an aspect often neglected by small companies.

Smart sourcing is the key to becoming a manufacturer of reliable world-class products, and Nocca needs to work with trusted component suppliers. But, in a world where quality is the final arbiter, the only way for a new company like Nocca to convince sceptics is to do whatever else may be required to deliver on that promise.

KEY TAKEAWAYS

Smart sourcing can make or break a business.

- Being smart about sourcing requires expertise and is crucial for realizing good product margins.
- Fully indigenizing a product is neither practical nor necessary; many components or raw materials may be available overseas at cheaper prices and at scale. What's more important is to do most of the high-quality work in India so that most of the value is captured locally.
- Moving sourcing away from China is not easy, but a start needs to be made sooner than later.

STARTER KIT

STEP 1: Do you operate in a market where competition or customer pressure makes it hard to increase prices, or are you among the lucky few (like Apple) where your brand or uniqueness allows you to charge premium pricing? If it's the former, then good sourcing is really the only way to make money. If it's the latter, sourcing helps to further improve margins. Being clear about where you stand is the first step.

STEP 2: Even for early-stage product startups, hiring sourcing experts is important. Apart from just making components or raw materials available at the right price and time, their relationships with suppliers can bring in new ideas as well as competitive insights from across the world.

STEP 3: As sales and production volumes grow, the sourcing team needs to work collaboratively with domestic companies in India to see if some of the crucial parts can be produced locally. Reducing dependence on China should be an equally important goal.

Notes

1. Yashdeep Kumar's interview with the authors.
2. Tapesh Sinha's interview with the authors.

6

Convincing the Sceptics

In the early hours of Sunday, on 5 July 2020, heavy rains, thunderstorm and lightning hit various parts of India. In Yamuna Nagar, Haryana, Dr A. V. S. Ravi woke up a worried man. [1] His forty-bed paediatric hospital had fourteen patients that night, and one of the babies was in critical care. The infant was being provided respiratory support and airway hydration and placed in a warmer for comfort.

Dr Ravi's home was in the same building as the hospital, and he woke up with a jolt at 2.30 a.m. when a power surge blew up all the electronic equipment around him. Within the span of a few minutes, his air conditioner, refrigerator, cable TV set-top box, laptop chargers, LED lights, stabilizers and CCTV cameras broke down. He looked out of his window. The hospital's LED sign had met the same fate. The phones no longer worked. He was struck by panic as he walked over to the hospital floor where the infant lay in critical care, connected to several electrical devices. He breathed a sigh of relief. The AIRVO 2 unit for respiratory support, the warmer and phototherapy units had all survived the surge. The infant was safe and healthy.

Critical care medical equipment is expensive, but it is not surprising Dr Ravi had willingly invested in them. Such equipment is invariably imported or made by multinational companies or their joint ventures in India. The AIRVO 2 was built by

Fisher & Paykel Healthcare, a New Zealand company that has been around since 1971, while the warmer and phototherapy units were the products of a Wipro-GE joint venture.

Dr Ravi had sworn by the dependability of such high-quality medical equipment after learning a lesson on reliability early on in his career. After completing his Short Service Commission with the Indian Navy and post-graduation at King George Medical College, Lucknow, he had started his Yamuna Nagar clinic in 1994, and then built an eight-bed hospital in 1997. During this early period, in an attempt to keep his costs low, he had bought a simple 'baby warmer' from a company in Saharanpur, Uttar Pradesh. But the warmer failed frequently as its quality was poor. That's when he decided he would only go for the best from thereon. Even though imported equipment was more expensive, especially for doctors and hospitals in small towns, Dr Ravi would wait until he had saved up enough money to buy such devices.

Could hospital owners like him ever come to trust medical equipment from Indian companies? Could such equipment become reliable as well as affordable? This was the challenge the IIT Kanpur Ventilator Consortium was faced with as it set out to build a world-class ventilator in the wake of the pandemic.

Indian hospitals and doctors buy ₹40,000 crore worth of medical equipment every year, but close to 80% is imported.[2] The numbers are similar for ventilators. Close to 5,500 of these devices are imported[3] each (non-Covid) year with global brands like Hamilton, Maquet, Drager, GE, Schiler, Philips and Mindray holding sway. But at an average price of ₹6.2 lakh per unit, many hospitals cannot afford to buy such expensive equipment. Interestingly, and in a scenario unique to India, over 700 refurbished ventilators are sold every year at an average price of ₹5.07 lakh.[3]

India undoubtedly needs affordable ventilators. Online platforms like IndiaMART or Avante host a whole array of refurbished multinational brands. But across the country, when Covid started spreading, the 48,000-odd ventilators were concentrated in just seven states – UP, Karnataka, Maharashtra, Tamil Nadu, West Bengal, Telangana, Kerala – leaving many states and hospitals with an inadequate number of ICU beds and ventilators. [4] Dr Sujata Mishra from Cuttack, Odisha, estimates that her city had over 100 nursing homes, but no more than seven had ICUs with working ventilators.[5]

As the task force, it was up to us to convert this challenge into an opportunity. We needed to assault this issue on three fronts:

1) Getting the 'reliable product–affordable price' equation right by designing for just the perfect balance
2) Making the product available nationwide and backed by good after-sales service
3) Building a relationship of trust and confidence with doctors

In late March, when the task force was being formed, the Nocca founders' initial ventilator design (Model V110) was an extremely simple one. It had just one mode (pressure control), and the user was expected to operate it using their own mobile phones. This design was in line with the specifications announced by Canada and the UK at the time to accelerate the development of ventilators for the pandemic. The Nocca founders were motivated by the idea of bringing out an affordable product as quickly as possible, and they estimated it could be done at a cost of ₹50,000. As they said, 'All we wanted to do was to prove [that] we could build and deploy a product like this for non-critical Covid cases. We weren't thinking about a business at all when we started.'

But the media somehow found out about the price, and a BBC News report[6] dated 31 March stated that 'the invasive ventilator being developed by Nocca Robotics will cost ₹50,000 rupees ($662)' created a stir. The founders were somewhat taken by surprise, but the price remained in public memory.

The V110 had a simple design. A month later, we learnt that NASA was introducing a ventilator on similar lines for their VITAL model. NASA announced on 1 May 2020 that it had received emergency use authorization from the Food and Drug Administration (FDA) for its new ventilator called VITAL (Ventilator Intervention Technology Accessible Locally).[7] But when the Ministry of Health and Family Welfare issued a series of guidelines about ventilator specifications in India, the designs had to be updated. Two more design iterations – V210 and V310 – followed soon after to meet the requirements. The V310 design, suitable for use by critical-care patients as well, was ready on 16 May.

But these significant design enhancements – which included a flow meter, a tablet and electronic control of oxygen flows – raised the price of the product. During its short-lived existence, the V210 was pegged at ₹150,000, while the final product, the V310, was expected to be priced at ₹350,000 (plus taxes). Although this would make it cheaper than most imported ventilators, the task force debated whether the prices could be driven even lower. But the higher cost of input components and the desire to stay away from the 'Nano trap' convinced us to stick with it. We remembered Tata's ambitious Nano project, which had failed because the low price of the vehicle made potential buyers suspicious about its quality.

Now that we had the answer to the 'reliable product–affordable price' equation, it was time to look at the logistics of making the ventilator available nationally once it was finally manufactured.

The question before us was similar to a talented batsman asking themselves at the early stages of their career whether they wanted to be a flashy T20 star like Chris Gayle or a seemingly boring but enduring cricketer like Rahul Dravid. Should we chase big Covid-specific government orders, or should we remain content as a steady long-term player with a sales presence across small and big cities across the country? Or should we do both?

After a massive government tender for ventilators was announced by HLL Lifecare Limited on 27 March 2020, Nocca filed a bid on 5 April. Winning even part of it would have been a big bounty for the team, but Nocca chose to play steady. The tender was opaque and confusing, and Nocca would find it hard to meet its deadlines if it wanted to deliver a high-quality product. It proved to be a good decision as we later found that some of our competitors had taken a shot at the tender and ended up with eggs on their faces!

With this in mind, the team had also started working on a sales and distribution strategy, with the medtech CEOs in the task force coming together to hire Vineet Kumar, the first full-time salesperson for the company. Vineet was tasked with appointing distributors and starting the process of building a potential market in smaller Indian cities. The task force ambitiously estimated that even without a big government order Nocca could use this distribution network to sell a large number of ventilators. When Vineet quickly appointed seventeen distributors in north and west India, and initial orders started coming in from places like Pune, Mumbai, Jalna (Maharashtra), Bijapur (Karnataka), Dahej (Gujarat) and Gurgaon (Haryana), these assumptions seemed to be holding true. The task force also began exploring a partnership with Aforeserve, a specialist service and repairs company with 4,000 employees across 350 Indian locations, to ensure that Nocca's ventilators could be installed and serviced as well.

There was another challenge. Nocca also needed a plan to convince doctors that their product was of high quality, affordable and easily available and serviceable if hospitals were to move away from imported ventilators. To do so, Nocca needed to build strong relationships with the medical community within a short period of time. Task force members began leveraging their experience to provide introductions to top doctors in Pune, Mumbai, Delhi and Gurgaon, whose responses were thankfully encouraging. There was also the hope that once the DGHS had tested the V310, and certified that it had all the features as laid out in government guidelines, this would boost the confidence in their ventilator in the medical community at large.

We now needed a catchy name for the V310 which would resonate with doctors. Hundreds of names were tossed around in our daily noon calls before we finally arrived at 'Noccarc' – a name that rhymed with 'Noah's Arc' which was instrumental in the continuation of life on earth after a devastating worldwide flood. It was planned that Nocca Robotics would remain the name of the company, while Noccarc would serve as the brand name for ventilators. It was important to make this distinction as the company still runs its original business of manufacturing robots for waterless cleaning of solar panels.

Although we had come up with a reliable product at an affordable price, and the medical community seemed be responding positively, there was a nagging feeling that a lot more was needed to be done for Nocca to be considered a serious player as a medical device manufacturer. There was also the ingrained belief among the medical community that foreign-made products are inevitably better. V. Raja, former President and CEO of GE Healthcare India, agrees. 'Most doctors are biased in favour of imported products. They see domestic equipment as inferior. At radiology clinics, I have seen doctors opt for latest imported equipment purely as a marketing gimmick.'[8]

So, we asked one of our medtech mentors Sanjay Banerjee, former managing director of Zimmer Biomet India, a global firm specializing in treating injuries to bones, joints and supporting soft tissues, how this could be resolved. He had three basic prescriptions: train doctors, train technicians and arrange for financing to purchase the equipment. Sanjay's former firm offered virtual training sessions to orthopaedic surgeons across

India, and he believed a similar initiative would help Nocca overcome the roadblock of a paucity of trained 'intensivists' (physicians who provide special care for critically ill patients) and technicians. Dr Sujata Mishra had similar advice for the Noccarc. 'You must reach out to important operative workshops and conferences, where leaders in the fields would demonstrate the equipment and vouch for its effectiveness and safety, which can only come from experience in using them.'

If Nocca does it right over the next few years, it can indeed become a torchbearer for India's domestic medical equipment industry. Dr Ravi says, 'If equipment is more affordable, we can procure more of them. Our country badly needs to design world-class equipment – if not alone, at least in collaboration as in other sectors.'

The beginnings of the product were rooted in a pandemic, but if Nocca aims high enough, it can easily scale to make Noccarc a story of Indian innovation and design at affordable prices, one of innovation under exceptional circumstances. However, the Nocca team will need to remember that there is no shortcut in the path to glory. To be a major global player to be reckoned with, they will have to establish the brand based on quality, dependability and service. Doctors cannot afford to take chances with their patients' lives.

But for this to happen, India desperately needs an effective, sensible and implementable regulatory regime that enables great, reliable medical devices to be built.

KEY TAKEAWAYS

Smart Indian entrepreneurs can create a market for high-quality domestic products.

- Doctors and hospitals in India are used to and comfortable with imported medical equipment due to bad experiences with domestic products.

- A multi-pronged strategy is required to change doctors' perceptions about the new generation of domestic medical devices: a great product that uses the best components and has undergone rigorous testing and certification; high-quality manufacturing standards; competitive pricing; a nationwide sales and distribution infrastructure and after-sales service network; and continuous training of doctors and equipment financing.
- Adequate funding is required to support these early efforts before the business becomes self-sustainable.

STARTER KIT

STEP 1: Pick a therapy-focused equipment (or a set of products) – from actual user discussions – that is in short supply or one with an imported counterpart that is inappropriate for Indian conditions. Assess the market. Can you see a ₹100-crore revenue and at least 15% EBITDA in three years? Only such scale and profitability will enable investments required to build reliable products and sustain doctors' confidence in them.

STEP 2: Develop robust plans that cover product design, sourcing, manufacturing, certification, branding, pricing, sales and distribution, service, training and customer financing. Don't make compromises while developing high-quality products; let yourself be guided on essential and desired features every step of the way by expert actual users. Unnecessary fancy features can be done away with but be careful that doctors don't get biased against you because of this.

STEP 3: Ensure adequate funding support and future visibility to meet cash gap for three years, while all these foundational investments are being made. Sustained efforts and stamina are required to survive this gruelling period. Within three years, the business should be cash positive and able to stand on its own feet if it has reached its targeted ₹100 crore revenue and 15% EBIDTA levels.

Notes

1. Dr A. V. S. Ravi's interview with the authors.
2. Akhter, Shahid, 'We Need to Come out of 80% Import Dependency in Medical Devices: Dr G.S.K. Velu.' ETHealthworld.com, 10 October 2018. https://health.economictimes.indiatimes.com/news/medical-devices/we-need-to-come-out-of-80-import-dependency-in-medical-devices-dr-g-s-k-velu/66149260.
3. Medical Buyer, 28 January 2020. https://www.medicalbuyer.co.in/ventilator-sales-take-a-hit-in-2019/.
4. Kapoor, Geetanjali et al. 'State wise Estimates of Current Hospital Beds, ICU Beds, and Ventilators.' Center for Disease Dynamics, Economics & Policy, 20 April 2020. https://cddep.org/publications/covid-19-in-india-state-wise-estimates-of-current-hospital-beds-icu-beds-and-ventilators/.
5. Dr Sujata Mishra's interview with the authors.
6. Biswas, Soutik. 'Coronavirus: India's Race to Build a Low-Cost Ventilator to Save Covid-19 Patients.' BBC News, 31 March 2020. https://www.bbc.com/news/world-asia-india-52106565.
7. Northon, Karen. 'Developed Ventilator Authorized by FDA for Emergency Use.' NASA, 30 April 2020. https://www.nasa.gov/press-release/nasa-developed-ventilator-authorized-by-fda-for-emergency-use.
8. V. Raja's interview with the authors.

7

The Regulatory Haze

On 3 October 1978, Doordarshan Calcutta reported the birth of the world's second and India's first test-tube baby, pseudo-named Durga. Indian physician-scientist Dr Subhas Mukherjee achieved the remarkable feat barely sixty-seven days after the birth of Louise Brown, the world's first test-tube baby.

A little less than three years later, on 19 June 1981, Dr Mukherjee committed suicide.

What had transpired in between makes for a sordid tale. Dr T. C. Anand Kumar, the leader of the team that gave birth to Harsha, India's first 'scientifically documented' IVF baby, lamented, 'As far as I am concerned, Mukherjee did reach great heights. His achievements in the biology of reproduction dwarf all other achievements in India in this field. Unfortunately, [the] ignorance of the medical fraternity, bureaucratic arrogance and vindictiveness led to the loss of one of our distinguished scientists. We also lost our claim to having been the first in the world to have succeeded in not only fertilizing human eggs in vitro but also having successfully cryopreserved the embryo, thawing it and leading to the birth of a healthy normal baby following the embryo's replacement into the mother's womb.'[1]

In addition to the malaises pointed out by Dr Anand Kumar, what contributed significantly to the humiliation and frustration of Dr Mukherjee was the lack of a regulatory framework under which his work could be documented, vetted and reported. Forty years later, today India's IVF industry is growing at 28% annually and is expected to be valued around ₹495 crore by 2022.[2]

Today, the exact number of babies born in India through various assisted reproductive technologies (ARTs) is not known. However, by the end of the century, nearly 4% of all the babies in the world will be born through ART.[3] India, with its high population, will feature prominently in that demographic.

Despite the phenomenal growth of ART in India, the regulatory framework to ensure the responsible use of such technology was extremely slow to catch up. It was only in 2005 that the National Guidelines for Accreditation, Supervision and Regulation of ART Clinics in India was promulgated by the Indian Council of Medical Research (ICMR) and the National Academy of Medical Sciences.[4] Although comprehensive, the guidelines were non-enforceable. Finally, in 2020, the Assisted Reproductive Technology (ART) Regulation Bill 2020 was passed by the Parliament. The bill is expected to usher in a new era for ART in India.

This kind of sluggishness in bringing out timely, effective and easy-to-navigate frameworks to help develop and market science- and technology-based services or products has been the Achilles' heel of the Indian regulatory establishment. What was true of ART has been true for medical devices as well. The chaos that we were to see soon around indigenous Covid-19 solutions highlighted this inadequacy in the most painful way.

Soon after the pandemic arrived in India, when ventilators were touted as one of the most effective management strategies for Covid-19 patients, on 4 April 2020, Prime Minister Modi directed the government committees that oversaw pandemic management to remove all roadblocks and rapidly scale up the production of domestic ventilators.[5] Several other officials emphasized the message, especially when it became apparent that importing ventilators was not an option.

Meanwhile, in Pune, the young Nocca team was racing against time to develop the prototype for the first version, V110. By 5 April 2020, it was ready.

At the beginning of the pandemic every country panicked and rushed to procure as many ventilators as possible as it was thought that COVID-19 pathology is like most other ARDS (Acute Respiratory Distress Syndrome) conditions and ventilators would be major lifesavers.[6] The rush to procure ventilators was such that in the US states were bidding against each other causing a massive price escalation.[7]

Presumably learning from this US experience, to prevent price escalations and state-level shortages, the Government of India decided to procure ventilators centrally. It had initiated its procurement process by the end of March 2020, and a government-owned company – HLL Lifecare Limited – was asked to procure critically needed supplies, including ventilators. The idea was to procure centrally and then distribute the machines to different states based on local requirements.

But the tender published by HLL on 27 March sent highly confusing signals to domestic manufacturers.[8] For, on the one hand, the specifications matched those of the most sophisticated imported ventilators, but on the other, the government had appealed to manufacturers to consider making them domestically. India has traditionally not been a major producer of such high-end medical devices. To expect Indian biomedical engineers to straightaway make such critical devices with the highest specifications, that too during a worldwide lockdown, was an optimistic ask, to put it mildly. The notice also asked suppliers to provide a list of all ventilators already deployed by them in major government hospitals in the last five years, a clause that would not be met by any Indian manufacturer other than the Mysuru-based Skanray, which had a production capacity of a few hundred ventilators per year.

Going by the notice, the scales seemed to be weighed in favour of imported ventilators. But on the flip side, the compliance requirements were simple, and seemed encouraging for new manufacturers. The tender only asked for basic compliance certification vis-à-vis electrical and general safety. It did not insist on the next higher level of certification for full EMI/EMC compliance; electromagnetic compatibility (EMC) and electromagnetic interference (EMI) together measure how well electrical devices can function while being hit with energy released from other electrical devices in the vicinity. EMI/EMC certification for a new device usually takes several months to attain.

Then again, the tender included other ambiguous requirements where it asked that the machine 'should be approved by a reputed national/international certifying agency'. It was not clear for what approval was being sought – design or manufacture or sales!

The tender was confusing not just for the Nocca founders who were developing the product, but also for our potential manufacturing partners. Some asked if our ventilator was approved by the ICMR or the DGHS, none of which are authorized to provide regulatory approval of medical devices in India. Others who were more knowledgeable asked us if our ventilator was approved by the Central Drugs Standard Control Organisation (CDSCO), a valid question, but strange, since medical devices are presently regulated in India by an agency that had originally been created to regulate drugs and cosmetics!

We needed to take a step back and think through this hazy picture of regulations. HLL was playing hard to get and would not give us a clear answer. Those proficient with medical devices within the task force were also not in the know.

This is when a breakthrough came from an unexpected quarter. As a member of the Confederation of Indian Industries' (CII) national committee on Biotechnology, Amitabha chanced upon an internal email with an attachment of a screenshot of another email. On 24 March, the Drug Controller General of

India, Dr V. G. Somani, had written to Dr P. D. Vaghela, the Secretary, Department of Pharmaceuticals, 'As desired by you, it is to inform you that presently no permission is required for manufacturing of ventilators under the Drugs and Cosmetics Act and Medical Device Rules. Therefore, those who are willing to come forward and manufacture ventilators may start the production to tackle the situation arising out of Covid-19 outbreak in public interest.'

Two things were immediately clear from this email. Firstly, even the top echelons of the government were groping for clarity about regulations surrounding the production of ventilators in India. Secondly, as strange as it sounds, as of late-March, there were no regulations that prevented anyone from manufacturing a ventilator and selling it to a hospital in India. This was an astounding revelation for all of us, considering that a ventilator is a critical life-saving device. However, at least one mystery was solved: we could go ahead and make a ventilator without prior approvals. How we wished this crucial information had been made known to stakeholders at large as part of the HLL tender!

The second mystery facing us was this: if there were no regulatory frameworks, how would it be possible for a certifying agency – national or international – to provide any certification? When we asked Anil Jauhri and M. G. Sathyendra, both associated with the Quality Council of India and the National Accreditation Board for Certification Bodies (NABCB), they confirmed that no agency in India was accredited to certify ventilators manufactured here.[9] Among the international systems, the two most popular ones are the European regulatory CE mark and the American FDA regulations. CE, or Conformitè Europëenne, is the European Union's mandatory conformity marking for regulating the goods sold there. It was possible to reach a notified body of Europe through its associates in India for CE certification or to approach USFDA directly since it does not have a system of third-party agencies. However, it would have taken at least six months to a year to obtain such certifications. In India, Skanray was the only manufacturer whose ventilators were certified by CE. However, it was designing a new ventilator model for Covid-19 patients and would have had to apply afresh for CE or FDA certification, making a launch during the lockdown unlikely. None of the other manufacturers we knew of had any certifications. That meant only imported ventilators would qualify for the tender. But because there was a worldwide shortage of ventilators, it would be impractical for the government to depend exclusively on imported models.

We were at a loss.

Anil Jauhari, who was previously CEO of NABCB, thought no other point in the HLL tender created as much confusion as the title itself: 'Tender Specifications for Ventilator'. Many types of devices can qualify as a ventilator; however, only the critical-care ventilator can serve Covid-19 patients. As no distinction had been made, and as the naïve ventilator manufacturer had no clue, every type of machine that could put out air at a high pressure was being touted as a ventilator. The media then disseminated news[10, 11, 12] of the development of each such machine by individuals and large corporates alike as the next big breakthrough, creating a perception that quality ventilators were available in the country in sufficient quantities to serve Covid-19 patients. But this was far from the truth.

It isn't just ventilators; X-ray machines have faced such regulatory haze for nearly four decades. X-ray machines aren't necessarily considered as dangerous today. However, in the 1980s, according to M. G. Sathyendra, who was then an officer at the Bureau of Indian Standards (BIS) in Mumbai, there were instances of operators receiving electric shocks from X-ray machines, and in one tragic case, a patient died when the tube head fell on him. This prompted the BIS to order mandatory certification of X-Ray machines according to a set of standards specified by it. To implement these promptly, BIS also rolled out standard operating procedures in 1986 that required all X-Ray clinics to be inspected by BIS officers, and the machines manufactured in India to be tested at the manufacturers' premises. This became impractical over the years as the number of both manufacturers and clinics increased. At the same time, the introduction of digital X-Ray machines made the 1986 rules obsolete. But the regulations remain the same today based on the 1986 norms, no matter how irrelevant they have become.

To put it simply, there are no regulatory provisions to date that ensure Indian manufacturers will make X-ray machines with internationally acceptable specifications.

A strict regulatory regime for the approval of the sale of medical devices is not an unnecessary burden. Rather, it is critical not only for patients but also for Indian manufacturers. But the existing casual approach towards good regulatory processes for medical devices is hurting Indian manufacturers. Imported brands from the US, Europe or East Asian countries possess internationally respected certifications and thus do not need to be tested and certified again in India. Since medical devices must be dependable, Indian hospitals and doctors readily trust and buy imported products with CE or FDA certification, as was the case with Dr Ravi of Yamuna Nagar.

Unless the expensive certifications from the FDA or CE can be obtained, Indian manufacturers can only earn the trust of Indian doctors and patients the hard way – through high-quality performance and reliability. But convincing doctors and hospitals can become much easier if an efficient, strict and transparent regulatory and certification regime is put in place, where the standards are defined and made relevant for India and are in sync with international standards. Only this can make 'Made in India' products credible.

Ideally, a medical device certification body that has several accredited laboratories throughout the country should be set up.

These labs should be able to test: (1) the technical parameters of a medical device; (2) its durability and reliability; and (3) the mechanical, electrical and electronic safety of the device. The whole process – from submitting the device for testing to getting the test data – should not take more than a month. Once the test results indicate that a machine is safe, reliable and as per specifications, the regulatory body should issue permission for sale within a week's time.

Had such a system been in place when the Nocca team took up their task in March, they would have known what to build from the very beginning and would not have had to constantly readjust their trajectory along the way. The V310 could have been developed earlier if the regulatory haziness had not slowed them down. Also, had a proper regulatory system been in place, so many controversial incidents with malfunctioning ventilators would not have been in the news further hurting the brand India.

KEY TAKEAWAYS

Regulatory haze is bad for 'Make in India'.

- India lacks a strict, but fair and transparent, regulatory framework for many medical devices.
- The absence of such a framework makes it hard for both manufacturers and the medical community.
- Indian products will gain credibility only with a regulatory framework that meets global standards while being relevant to the country's needs.
- There should ideally be a separate medical device certification body with many accredited laboratories across the country.

Notes

1. Kumar, Anand T. C. 'Architect of India's First Test-Tube Baby: Dr Subhas Mukherji.' (16 January 1931 to 19 July 1981). *Current Science* 72. No. 7. (10 April 1997). https://www.currentscience.ac.in/Downloads/article_id_072_07_0526_0531_0.pdf.
2. Banker, Manish. '41 Years of IVF – The Revolution of Assisted Reproductive Technology!' ETHealthworld.com, 25 July 2019. https://health.economictimes.indiatimes.com/news/industry/41-years-of-ivf-the-revolution-of-assisted-reproductive-technology/70380646.
3. Ibid.
4. Murthy, Laxmi, Subramanian, Vani. 'ICMR guidelines on Assisted Reproductive Technology: Lacking in Vision, Wrapped in Red Tape.' *Indian Journal of Medical Ethics*, 4. No. 3 (30 November 2016). https://ijme.in/articles/icmr-guidelines-on-assisted-reproductive-technology-lacking-in-vision-wrapped-in-red-tape/.
5. 'PM Modi Meets Covid-19 Task Force, Urges Empowered Groups to Ensure Availability of Essential Healthcare.' TimeNowNews.Com. Updated 4 April 2020. https://www.timesnownews.com/india/article/pm-modi-meets-covid-19-task-force-urges-empowered-groups-to-ensure-availability-of-essential-healthcare/573809.
6. Netland, Torbjørn. 'A Better Answer to the Ventilator Shortage as the Pandemic Rages On.' World Economic Forum, 3 April 2020. https://www.weforum.org/agenda/2020/04/covid-19-ventilator-shortage-manufacturing-solution/.
7. Voytko, Lisette. 'Cuomo Says Ventilators Cost $50,000 up from $20,000 as States Compete for the Devices.' *Forbes*, 30 March 2020. https://www.forbes.com/sites/lisettevoytko/2020/03/30/cuomo-says-ventilators-cost-50000-up-from-20000-as-states-compete-for-the-devices/?sh=1f201bc78b3f.
8. Manek, Shreedhar. 'Favouritism and Fake Certifications Mar India's Ventilator Procurement.' *Ken*, 5 May 2020. https://the-ken.com/story/ventilator-procurement-problems/.
9. Mr Anil Jauhri and Mr M. G. Sathyendra's interview with the authors.

10. Panday, Amit. 'Covid-19: Mahindra's Indigenously Developed Ventilator to Cost Less than ₹7,500.' *Mint*, 26 March 2020. https://www.livemint.com/companies/news/coronavirus-m-m-ready-with-ventilator-prototype-to-cost-less-than-rs-7-500-11585228399566.html.
11. 'Coronavirus: ISRO to Design Ventilators, Oxygen Canisters, Make Hand Sanitisers.' *Mint*, 29 March 2020. https://www.livemint.com/news/india/coronavirus-isro-to-design-ventilators-oxygen-canisters-make-hand-sanitisers-11585472246736.html.
12. 'Coronavirus: IIT-Roorkee Develops Prana-Vayu, a Low-Cost Ventilator.' *Hindu*, 3 April 2020. https://www.thehindu.com/news/national/coronavirus-iit-roorkee-develops-prana-vayu-a-low-cost-ventilator/article31252339.ece.

8

Games People Play

On 5 May 2020, the reputed online business news portal the *Ken* reported, 'Favouritism and fake certifications mar India's ventilator procurement'.[1] The story revealed how an Indian ventilator manufacturer had been claiming its products to be 'FDA and CE compliant'. However, the certificates had been issued by a certain Unitas Certification Services, a web-based company whose net asset as per its company filings report was £1 ($1.25). Yet, the ventilator manufacturer had claimed on its Facebook page way back in July 2018 that its ventilators and manufacturing facility to be FDA and CE compliant.

When the *Ken*'s report started to make the rounds within relevant government corridors and WhatsApp groups run by ventilator manufacturers, the Facebook post was removed, but the thumbnail could still be viewed online. It was clear that the certifications procured by the manufacturer – at least at that point – had been issued by web-based companies whose standard operating procedures were shady at best. According to industry insiders, loopholes within Indian laws allowed such entities to operate since there is no law in India against setting up a certification body. Any entity can claim to be a certification agency in India. There is no need to demonstrate competence in certifying a range of products.

Certificates from an agency other than the USFDA (US Food and Drug Administration) itself that say a product is USFDA compliant mean nothing. Understandably, no other agency is entitled to use the USFDA logo. Not only that, the USFDA does not actually certify a product that is to be sold in India, rather, it approves a product for sale in the USA. Sadly enough, even seasoned medical practitioners and senior administrators at hospitals did not understand these nuances and were taken in by these claims.

Not surprisingly, media reports from Gujarat[2] and Mumbai[3] soon revealed that locally manufactured ventilators from at least two companies were of poor quality and not fit for Covid management but had been installed in hospitals only to be rejected later amid huge hue and cry. These machines were perhaps not rigorously tested by the manufacturers or by competent third-party agencies that were qualified to test an ICU ventilator. Thankfully, the government sensed trouble and realized the problems that could come from procuring any and every ventilator for installation in Covid wards.

This is when the Ministry of Health and Family Welfare came up with a solution which, although temporary, was better than nothing. We learnt on 16 May that a committee of experts had been set up under the DGHS and tasked with rigorously evaluating all ventilators that were to be deployed at hospitals.

It is clear that the absence of a rigorous certification process hurts Brand India. The failure of some of these 'Made in India' machines further propagated the stereotype that Indian medical devices were not reliable. The IIT-K task force had to navigate such minefields carefully. Our competitors were making big claims and walking away with massive government orders. We also had to watch out for the games played by our competitors during these months, and here, task force member Pavan Choudary, who is not just a successful CEO but also an author and a public intellectual, had sound advice for us every time we faced a situation involving a competitor's dirty tricks.

Many of India's large industry bodies were actively involved in brainstorming solutions since the beginning of the pandemic. At one such meeting, a large Indian corporation that was in the arena for making ventilators tried to run down local innovators by questioning their ability to rise to the occasion. Much to everyone's amusement, the chairperson – a reputed doctor – shot down the company's product. On another occasion, a junior executive from the same company sent a mail to the Nocca founders expressing interest in a partnership and asked for the product design. We wisely ignored the mail.

It was not just the larger companies that were playing such games. A mid-tier medical equipment manufacturer wanted to grab a share of the government tender but knew nothing about ventilators. They partnered with one of the IITs in order to develop one. The design was good, but they were unable to globally source the components that were required to manufacture this design. So, they began talking to us in mid-April under the pretext of becoming a manufacturing partner for the V310. A week later, and after a few meetings where they were briefed about our design, they used a flimsy excuse – that the other IIT was 'unwilling to release them from the contract' – to walk away. Quite clearly, they had engaged us only to take a closer look at our design that was based on available components during a volatile supply environment.

Yet another company, a reputed mid-size medical device manufacturer, approached us in late-April claiming that they had orders in hand and were keen to partner with Nocca Robotics to produce and supply the V310 ventilators since they did not have a product of their own. Thankfully, we had also learned to be cautious by this time. We discovered a month later that they actually had a product of their own and had been in the same room as Nocca Robotics trying to get a nod for their product from the DGHS panel. From what we know, they had failed even after four attempts to get an approval for their product. We thanked our stars that we had not shared our actual design with them.

Members of our task force are all celebrated professionals in their respective domains, and most of them have good reputations in the medical devices or innovation arena. From March to May, as the news media regularly reported the efforts of various entities around the country towards making ventilators, they would often reach out to our task force members for their insights and views. During such discussions, the journalists would narrate some of the shady things that they had seen or heard. Very often, multiple members of our task force would be approached by journalists for such stories. This helped us stay updated about the shortcuts many of our competitors were taking.

Simultaneously, our sourcing team had built a good network of relationships with several medical device component suppliers. These suppliers would sometimes provide insights about the quantities of components being imported by other ventilator manufacturers, or about sourcing challenges being faced by them. This helped us get a closer view of market realities and clear out some of the hype around our competitors' tall claims in circulation at the time.

While the experienced mentors in the task force helped us anticipate and prepare for such competitive games, our energies remained focused on ensuring that we build a very good product that would get early approval from the DGHS. We would get there soon, but only after encountering some minor heartbreaks on our way.

KEY TAKEAWAYS

Innovators cannot afford to ignore competitors.

- Be prepared for the fact that competitors, big or small, will adopt the principle of 'all's fair in love and war'.
- Innovators are often unprepared to deal with the tricks and deceit of competitors.
- Experienced mentors can help innovators navigate such minefields.

STARTER KIT

STEP 1: As part of their targets or key result areas (KRAs), ask your sales teams to provide regular structured feedback on the competition's activities by talking to distribution partners and customers. The supply chain or sourcing teams should be asked to do the same by getting information on your competitors' buying patterns and quantities.

STEP 2: Develop a good network of relationships with business and trade media that covers your industry. Journalists can provide insights that may validate what you may be hearing from your sales and supply chain teams or could offer totally fresh discoveries.

STEP 3: Create an advisory board of experienced mentors who know the industry well. Very often, they can just make a few phone calls to the right people – customers, trade and so on – and get the information you need. Not just that, they can help with troubleshooting and offer good advice when you are faced with competitors who don't play straight.

Notes

1. Manek, Shreedhar. 'Favouritism and Fake Certifications Mar India's Ventilator Procurement.' *Ken*, 5 May 2020. https://the-ken.com/story/ventilator-procurement-problems/.
2. 'Locally-Made Ventilators Not Good Enough Say Guj Officials.' *Week*, 18 September 2019. https://www.theweek.in/wire-updates/national/2020/05/18/bes5-gj-virus-ventilators.html.
3. Shukla, Archana. 'Mumbai Hospitals Return 81 Ventilators Made by AgVa-Maruti on Non-Performance.' CNBCTV18.com, 30 June 2020. https://www.cnbctv18.com/healthcare/mumbai-hospitals-return-81-ventilators-made-by-agva-maruti-on-non-performance-6227951.htm.

9

Agnipariksha

The entire task force was waiting for the message with bated breath. It arrived at 5.48 p.m. on 19 June 2020. 'HLL demo all clear,' announced Nikhil on the WhatsApp group. The group immediately lit up with congratulatory messages. The young Nocca team had gone in for the *agnipariksha* (ordeal by fire) and come out unscathed. The DGHS committee report issued that evening confirmed that the V310 had met all the requirements for the essential features laid out in the government's procurement specifications. In just eighty-two days, Nocca had accomplished the unthinkable. It had taken their concept of an ICU ventilator through manufacturing and the all-important regulatory approvals.

The DGHS approval was by no means the only test the V310 would have to pass. After the DGHS approval, the next agnipariksha would be with doctors, hospitals and their evaluation committees. We had been preparing ourselves to jump over all these hurdles ever since the task force was first created on 29 March and the ventilator was being designed and developed.

As early as 5 April, the task force had helped Nocca prepare for its first real test by developing the first iteration, the V110, which could be submitted as a bid to HLL (Hindustan Lifecare Ltd). Our bid proposed two models: (1) the V110, which was ready and offered as a pragmatic model for India's urgent needs but did not satisfy one essential specification (that is, regulation by volume control mode); and (2) the V210, which was fully compliant to specifications, but was under development at the time. We declared as much in our bid document.

The V110 model was based on precedents from the UK and Canada where the governments had announced specifications for emergency ventilators that did not mandate a volume control mode of regulation. From a practical standpoint, sensors that were needed to make ventilators with such a mode were not available. We had hoped that, just like in the UK and Canada, India would also relax that criteria. But it never did because a ventilator without the volume control mode is not exactly fit to manage Covid-19 patients. In hindsight, we were glad we submitted the V210 as well, for it had this mode built into its specifications.

Like nervous students awaiting exam results, the entire task force was anxious to hear how we would fare in this first test. Then on 16 April, the Nocca team received an email from HLL that said both the V110 and V210 could not be recommended as they did not meet the essential technical features (ETFs). This decision was based on the documents submitted by us.

We were baffled. We knew the V110 did not meet the ETFs, but we were at our wits' end when it came to understanding why the V210 did not. Our submission had clearly spelt out that the V210 was under development in line with the HLL specifications. As a documentation exercise, we had declared full compliance. Why did we then not pass the test?

It was only when the *Ken* reported on various issues with the government's ventilator procurement[1] that the mystery was solved. The 5 April Nocca submission was based on specifications HLL had placed in the public domain on 31 March. However, in the interim, a few more criteria were added that were made public only on 18 April. The V210 was disqualified based on specifications that were not even publicly known at the time of submitting the bid, or even when the verdict was announced on 16 April! The goalposts had been shifted midway – even as we were preparing for one kind of agnipariksha, the evaluator decided to score us on a different one.

The Nocca team did not give up. They began developing a more advanced version, the V310, that would not only satisfy all essential and desirable procurement specifications but would also have additional features. The first design for the V310 was ready by 24 April, and the team was confident enough to inform HLL. While we kept waiting for a meeting invitation for several weeks, the team kept improving the design. By the time, we were finally invited for a meeting with HLL on 16 May, the V310 was fully ready and in full glory – with both pressure and volume control modes and a new user interface. But alas, the HLL meeting was only for them to tell us about yet another change in policy. All companies would now need to demonstrate their product to a DGHS technical committee in New Delhi.

This became our new goal.

While we waited for the DGHS demo to be scheduled, the V310 successfully cleared a test for compliance to the IEC 60601-1 standard on 27 May. The International Electrotechnical Commission (IEC) prepares and publishes international standards for all electrical, electronic and related technologies.[2] By clearing IEC 60601-1 test at the NABL-accredited Swen Konformity Lab in Pune, the V310 was shown to conform with the 'General Requirements for Basic Safety and Essential Performance'.

On 8 June, the Nocca founders received an unexpected call from HLL inviting them for a demo at 5 p.m. the same day at Nirman Bhawan, New Delhi. No advance notice, just a call out of the blue. Serendipitously, the Nocca team happened to be in Delhi that day, being en route to Lucknow to provide a demonstration of the ventilator at King George's Medical

University (KGMU) Hospital and Sanjay Gandhi Postgraduate Institute of Medical Sciences (popularly known as SGPGI) Hospital. They scrambled to change their plans and were able to reach Nirman Bhawan in time.

The purpose of the meeting was to demonstrate the machine's features, including its delivery of FiO_2 (Fraction of inspired Oxygen). Most Covid-19 patients need a higher concentration of oxygen than the 21% that's present in normal atmospheric air, and so oxygen is supplemented to the ventilator. The DGHS committee wanted to check if FiO_2 levels could be adjusted independent of other parameters. When the Nocca team reached the venue, they realized that they were supposed to carry their own oxygen cylinder to demonstrate the FiO_2 delivery features! They were asked to return since the feature could not be demonstrated. However, the DGHS team supervising the demo was competent and compassionate and gave the Nocca team excellent tips to improve their model.

The next email from HLL arrived on 11 June asking for a demonstration of the further modified V310 at Nirman Bhawan within the next ten days. This time, the email categorically asked that we bring our own oxygen cylinder for the demo. No more surprises. The V310 got a clean chit on 19 June and the team of DGHS doctors certified it the same day as meeting all the ETFs. They recommended that before routine clinical use, the ventilator should be clinically validated, and that appropriate certificates and approvals must be obtained.

Wild 'virtual' celebrations broke out on our WhatsApp group when the news was shared. Emoji hugs were exchanged, virtual champagne bottles cracked open and firecrackers burst. The Nocca team had successfully passed the first agnipariksha.

The DGHS' recommendations for obtaining clinical validation were reasonable. The V310 could do what we claimed it could do and had satisfied the criteria set by India. But it was still important to ensure it worked properly on a patient. No good doctor would allow a machine as critical as an ICU ventilator to be used on a patient before an independent agency had certified it to be fit for ICU usage, as well as safe and dependable. The demo report from the DGHS committee, and the safety and reliability test reports from Swen Konformity thus set up the stage for testing the V310 on patients.

Dr Prachee Sathe, Director-ICU, at Ruby Hall Clinic, Pune, knew the V310 closely, and had been guiding the Nocca team from the beginning. When the team had requested her for guidance as they were working on their design, she had made a very pertinent comment: 'You should know that a patient suffering from ARDS is sometimes kept on a ventilator for weeks, if not months. How do you know that the machine can operate non-stop for such a long time?' Anticipating that the V310 would soon get the DGHS nod, Dr Sathe had offered to set up an endurance test for the ventilator. On 1 June, the Nocca team placed one machine at the critical care unit of Ruby Hall, where it ran non-stop for twenty-four days and a detailed log for this entire period was maintained. The V310 had successfully cleared the endurance test.

When we obtained the approved DGHS demo report on 19 June, the team went back to Dr Sathe and requested her to help with patient testing. She examined the test reports and then started planning for the patient testing. One of Dr Sathe's younger colleagues agreed to have the machine tested on himself as a healthy volunteer. Only after Dr Sathe was fully satisfied with the outcome did she put a critically ill pneumonia patient with respiratory failure on the V310. A team of experienced doctors was ready on site, while an imported ventilator stood by as back-up just in case the V310 failed to do its job.

But the V310 succeeded. In fact, it performed admirably. On 26 June, Dr Sathe certified the V310 fit to be used in the ICU.

The second agnipariksha had been passed just as we hit the ninety-day mark.

On 29 June, the machine was tested by two leading hospitals in Delhi–NCR – Medanta and Artemis – where it performed well. The icing on the cake was the test report from the Delhi Cantonment Base Hospital of Indian Armed Forces we received a few weeks later. The doctors at the Base Hospital who had evaluated the V310 gave it a rave review. With some minor modifications, they believed the machine could compete with any imported brand.

And this is how we passed yet some more agniparikshas.

As these positive results kept coming in, the team, buoyed with confidence, felt ready to enter the market. It had made good headway with the smaller private hospitals across the country, but the big government order via HLL remained elusive. In hindsight, the task force realized it could have done a few things differently to secure that order. Task force member and policy expert Pavan Choudary believes we didn't have the right kind of expertise to access and engage the government, that our knowledge about the government's purchase process was not adequate, and that we didn't have boots on the ground to facilitate the purchase. We were also conservative in that we delayed our public relations until the product was fully ready and certified.

Nonetheless, the V310 had passed the most stringent of tests and was ready to contribute to the cause of an 'Atmanirbhar Bharat'. We had been preparing since April for the mass scale manufacture of Nocaarc V310. Most of the groundwork had been completed, and it was now time to step on the gas.

KEY TAKEAWAYS

Innovation needs sunshine, not darkness.

- Critical medical equipment needs to pass several tests before being deployed.

- Lack of transparency and shifting goalposts make it harder to prepare for these tests.
- A strict but clear regulatory regime, coupled with a transparent certification process, will encourage local innovators to work towards an Atmanirbhar Bharat.

STARTER KIT

STEP 1: Bring on board a regulatory expert, possibly a consultant, early in your journey of product design and development. This person should not only help lay out a clear roadmap for all the approvals and certifications required, but also guide the team in implementing the same.

STEP 2: If the government is likely to be a big buyer of your product or service, it is vital to have an experienced person well versed in government purchase processes, including the recently announced 'Startup Runway' on the Government eMarketplace (GeM).

STEP 3: While it may appear premature to start publicizing your product before it is fully ready, there is definite merit in creating some visibility in advance so that buying decision makers and influencers do not view your product as unknown and of uncertain origins.

Notes

1. Manek, Shreedhar. 'Favouritism and Fake Certifications Mar India's Ventilator Procurement.' *Ken*, 5 May 2020. https://the-ken.com/story/ventilator-procurement-problems/.
2. 'International Electrotechnical Commission.' Wikipedia. Wikimedia Foundation, [Edited on] 9 December 2020. https://en.wikipedia.org/wiki/International_Electrotechnical_Commission.

10

Atmanirbhar Bharat: No Shortcuts

It was a Sunday in mid-April. The workload that particular day was not very intense, and the task force for once was not in firefighting mode. The discussions that day took a more philosophical turn. Always the incurable optimist, Amitabha declared 'At our incubator, we now have more than fifteen medtech startups. Clearly, young people are seeing a future in this line of business.' Before we could start revelling in these stories of success, the ever-pragmatic Sanjiv Verma – our manufacturing expert – gently steered the conversation towards the nuts and bolts of getting our product manufactured well, and at scale.

Srikant then narrated the Indian manufacturing experience of one of his IIT Kanpur classmates, Sanjeev Maddila. US-based Sanjeev has always had a natural soft corner for India. His consultancy firm helps large global corporations reduce costs of manufacturing, sourcing and distribution. When they ask for advice, he often tries to steer his clients to do more in or with India. Just over a decade ago, he persuaded a large American multinational medical technologies firm ($7 billion in revenues at that time) to explore Indian options when they were trying to source high-precision machined (stainless steel) components and medical-grade moulded plastic. Sanjeev took the company's representatives to potential suppliers in Delhi–NCR, Chennai and Coimbatore, but they went away unimpressed, compared to how they had felt during their recces in China and Singapore. Even though the Indian factories they visited were spick and span, the surroundings were not. Sanjeev recalls that it was a rude shock for some of the visitors, especially compared to Shenzhen, 'where they could see ten factories in a row'.[1] Even though labour costs in India were low, mechanized manufacturing made overall costs in China more competitive.

We were aware that many things had changed in the past decade, and more so especially during the pandemic. We were observing how India was quickly moving from having a near-zero manufacturing capacity for personal protective equipment (PPE) to becoming a significant player in a short period. By early-May, media reports were already announcing that with a capacity of 1.5 lakh units per day, India had become the second largest PPE producer in the world.[2] On the back of this achievement, and exports to other countries including the US and the UK, the government proclaimed that India's medical equipment industry had become self-sufficient.

We wondered whether this 'Mission Accomplished' announcement was premature, given that the pandemic presented India with only a short-term opportunity. Could such ramp-up of PPE production be sustained once there was no more pandemic-induced demand? After all, during the pandemic, the government itself acquired and distributed 1.28 crore PPEs for free within India and sold another 23 lakh units in exports.[3] Could various government agencies come together to orchestrate such support for medical equipment during normal times?

For Noccarc V310 to become a celebrated international medical device brand, it was critical to ensure it was manufactured to the exact specifications of the excellent product design developed by the team. The initial idea was that we needed to choose one or two manufacturing partner(s) for this purpose. The task force had begun scanning the Indian manufacturing landscape in early-April itself for high-quality partnerships to produce the Noccarc ventilator on a large scale.

This search picked up momentum in mid-April when Sanjiv Verma joined the effort. There were several promising conversations with large and mid-sized companies, but many dropped out because of one reason – they were all attracted by the possibility of big government orders during the pandemic. They kept waiting, and when it was clear that the government will no longer be placing big ventilator orders after the initial order of 49,000 units[4] announced in early April while exports were banned, their interest waned. We concluded that besides the usual '3L' issue of land, labour and legislation, what is really needed to make Atmanirbhar Bharat a success is a sharp increase in domestic demand. In many categories of capital equipment such as medical devices, governments – both centre and state – as big buyers have a key role to play.

The Atmanirbhar Bharat project is made of various elements and pillars, and is subject to multiple interpretations, but its underlying aim is simple: for India to be a bigger, better and stronger economy on the world stage. Using the PPE production success as an optimistic example for Atmanirbhar Bharat is tempting, but risky in the absence of an assured source of continuous product sales. There cannot be any shortcuts here.

Ador Powertron, a Pune-based industrial electronics company, was one of several companies that reached out to Nocca on 6 April, when the media hype about ventilators had gone sky-high. Their real interest was in bidding for the large government tender by putting forth the Noccarc V310 as the product they would manufacture. At one stage, when we began exploring a partnership with a public sector undertaking (PSU) to jointly bid for the government tender, we suggested to Ador that they focus on the regular market. They quickly lost interest. This wasn't surprising. For medical equipment manufacturers, it is a chicken-or-egg conundrum: should they look towards a large and assured sales pipeline first, or should they invest in manufacturing infrastructure first?

The sharpest answer to this question came from Sanjiv Verma, formerly associated with Baxter India. 'There is very little incentive in the Indian market for a progressive Indian manufacturer to embark on developing any capital-intensive medical equipment.' The underlying reasons are simple. Over 60% Indians pay for surgeries out of their own pockets and their budgets are small. Small budgets mean inexpensive treatments; therefore, hospitals cannot afford to use top-quality equipment, and this means there are no buyers for such equipment. There are only two ways to break this logjam. One is for the government to substantially increase its investment in healthcare infrastructure and increase demand for good equipment. The other way is for health insurance to cover much larger sections of our population. Sanjiv argues that, at just 20% penetration, India is among the least-insured countries when it comes to health insurance. If insurance pays for treatment, hospitals will have the ability to invest in better equipment. Insurance expansion will take time, and so, if India must attain Atmanirbhar status with respect to medical equipment, the only 'god' that matters is the government.

Unfortunately, the government has not always provided its blessings, as the power equipment industry once discovered. Atul Mishra, MD of consulting firm e-Gateway, and an experienced veteran of this industry since the 1980s, has been witness to this tragedy.[5] After their initial bias towards multinationals (GE, Siemens, Westinghouse and some Japanese companies) until the late 1970s, the government strongly backed Indian power equipment industry for the next two decades. A BHEL–Siemens partnership was structured, several mid-sized Indian companies making boilers and turbines emerged, and the main government buyers NTPC and state electricity boards were instructed to buy from these Indian companies. So far so good.

But as the century turned, China upgraded its four large state-owned power equipment companies to prepare themselves for a massive expansion of power generation capacity to a million megawatts by 2010. With state support, Chinese manufacturers got sudden scale and cost benefits. From 2006 onwards, as India began boosting its own power generation capacity, many Indian IPPs (independent power producers) started purchasing equipment from China at prices 20% lower than what Indian suppliers could offer. India's power generation capacity rapidly moved up to 375,000 MW, but Indian equipment manufacturers got left behind. With a surplus power of 75,000 MW today, they are unlikely to get any business in the near future. This tragedy could have been averted had the government stepped in at the right time to provide support like the Chinese government did to local manufacturers.

For the medical equipment industry to avoid this fate, the government needs to back it strongly through a beneficial tariff structure that incentivizes local manufacturing (for example, zero duty on component imports), ensuring that government procurement especially at prominent hospitals like the All India Institute of Medical Sciences (AIIMS) are not biased towards imported brands, and by instituting equipment certification standards that are relevant to India yet world-class. The harder bit, and this is what will create a long-term foundation as China did, is to scale up investments in healthcare infrastructure. The more well-equipped hospitals across the country, the greater will be the demand for high-quality medical equipment. This can be the trigger for India to become a global centre for affordable medical equipment.

India is now considered a major global supplier of high-quality automotive components and engineering goods. This wasn't always so, and nor is the government responsible for this transformation. Industry participants instead attribute this transformation to a second god – a large corporation with critical mass that raises the bar. It was Maruti Suzuki that brought scale as well as a quality mindset to this industry. Nirmal Jain, director of Solo Manufacturing and partner at Precicast, has witnessed the transformation of the industry since the 1980s.[6] During the pre-Maruti era, he supplied components to Kelvinator for their Avanti moped. He says, 'Kelvinator first discussed price, and then quality.' On the other hand, the conversation with Maruti Suzuki, to whom he has been supplying since 1990, has always begun with quality and timely deliveries and then gone on to price. He attributes the quality-related changes to the supplier eco-system that Maruti Suzuki created. This has helped his business compete across the world, 'We export to Fiat Italy and deliver the parameters they want. We are the sole supplier of connecting rods for a range of Honda generator sets that are manufactured in India and exported globally.' What pleased Nirmal the most is that 'India makes engineering and auto components that are better than what the Chinese make, even though they have greater volumes.'

For the medical equipment industry, it is unlikely that an industry flagbearer like Maruti Suzuki will suddenly appear to transform its fortunes. The onus therefore rests on the government to create demand so that private investments in equipment design and manufacturing can follow. Medtech expert Yashdeep Kumar, who is Vice President at the Global Innovations Program of the $14.9 billion medical technology giant Stryker Corporation, is clear that India 'first needs to fix the customer buying power. The government, both central and state, as a big buyer, has a key role to play in ensuring scale. Without scale, neither MNCs nor local entrepreneurs will be interested.'[7]

At a time when many countries are resetting their relationship with China, India now has a window of opportunity. Indian diplomats – traditionally not focused on trade and commerce – are now at the frontlines pitching to global companies to invest in India. Rahul Chabbra, Secretary of Economic Relations at the Ministry of External Affairs and one of the diplomats tasked with evangelizing Atmanirbhar Bharat, describes this opportunity succinctly: 'Government wants manufacturing here, but do so to supply the world.'[8] Ajay Bisaria, the Indian High Commissioner to Canada, has already reached out to over fifty Canadian companies, inviting them to India as an investment destination. He sees the companies diversifying their risks by moving from 'only China' to 'China plus one'.[9]

India thus needs to win this in two stages. At stage one, we need to be the 'plus one' country that companies prefer to locations like Vietnam, and secure that initial investment. Thereafter, if companies have good investment and manufacturing experience, stage two will kick in, and such companies may fully shift their investments from China. In every industry, including medical devices, India can make this a slam dunk if our domestic market and demand can be raised to such levels that it would be foolish for a global company to not manufacture here.

What will make Atmanirbhar Bharat a success is a combination of greater local demand, increased investment and a better manufacturing policy environment. Large private companies, PSUs and SMEs will all gain from this. This needs to play out over the next decade. There can be no shortcuts.

KEY TAKEAWAYS

Atmanirbhar Bharat will succeed only if government buys locally manufactured products.

- In India, the central and state governments are among the biggest buyers of many kinds of capital equipment, such as medical equipment.
- Domestic demand will grow if the government provides support by buying locally manufactured products and incentivizing local production.
- If domestic demand is strong, even global companies will come here for their manufacturing needs.
- Growth of manufacturing activity and investments will be the path to an Atmanirbhar Bharat.

Notes

1. Sanjeev Maddila's interview with the authors.
2. 'India Becomes World's 2nd Largest PPE Kit Producer in Just Two Months; Develops World's First Reusable PPE Suit.' *Swarajyamag*, 7 May 2020. https://swarajyamag.com/insta/india-becomes-worlds-2nd-largest-ppe-kit-producer-in-just-two-months-develops-world-first-reusable-ppe-suit.
3. Press Information Bureau. 'India Marches Ahead with "Atmanirbhar Bharat."' 14 August 2020. https://pib.gov.in/PressReleasePage.aspx?PRID=1645751.
4. Maheshwari, Dhairya. 'Ordered 1.7 Crore PPEs, 49,000 Ventilators, Health Ministry Reveals.' IndiaTV News, 9 April 2020. https://www.indiatvnews.com/news/india/ordered-1-7-crore-ppes-49-000-ventilators-health-ministry-reveals-coronavirus-606064.
5. Atul Mishra's interview with the authors.
6. Nirmal Jain's interview with the authors.
7. Yashdeep Kumar's interview with the authors.
8. Rahul Chabbra's interview with the authors.
9. Ajay Bisaria's interview with the authors.

11

A 'Make in India' Formula that Works

Chirag Gala, Sanjiv Verma, Nikhil Kurele and Harshit Rathore. The manufacturer, the manufacturing mentor and the ventilator designers respectively. The first desperately wanted to study at an IIT but could not, the second graduated from IIT Kharagpur forty-nine years ago, and the last two more recently – just four years ago – from IIT Kanpur. Fate brought them together to create a new 'Make in India' formula with the ventilator project and to show that it really works.

As a kid, Chirag Gala was fascinated by gadgets. At school one day, as his science teacher described a solar cooker to his class, Chirag raised his hand and offered to make one. The teacher, taken aback, laughed off his offer in disbelief. A week later, Chirag walked into school, cooker in hand, and went on to make idlis. His solar cooker is still on display at the A. H. Wadia High School in Mumbai. Chirag dreamt of going to IIT and was among the best students at the Vidyasagar Classes, a well-known coaching centre in Mumbai for competitive entrance exams. But to his eternal regret, he couldn't take the IIT joint entrance exam (the JEE) because of a wedding in the family. He eventually went to a local engineering college in Mumbai and spent his spare time at the medical equipment factory his dad and uncle ran together. An MBA followed, and soon after, in 2009, he set up his own venture – AVI Healthcare.

Starting as a distributor for an Italian brand of neo-natal ventilators, Chirag's inventive mind then conceptualized a 'transport incubator' that is used to provide a warm environment while transporting babies by road or air to an ICU or a hospital, for which he would win the ET Power of Ideas prize of ₹5 lakh in 2014. He went on to develop a few more neo-natal products, such as infantometers, warmers and phototherapy units.

But for all his talent and resourcefulness, Chirag unfortunately ran into the same troubles that plague SMEs in India: lack of funds, an inability to attract high-quality talent, and no access to cutting-edge technologies. These bottlenecks kept AVI Healthcare revenues to below ₹10 crore even after eleven years of operation.

Sanjiv Verma, who led all manufacturing partnership discussions for the task force, is a very unusual IITian. Unlike other IIT graduates of the 1970s who would fly off to the US right after college, his entire 1971 batch from Kharagpur was grounded in India because of the India-Pakistan war. Thus, the US's loss became a gain for Indian manufacturing, as Sanjiv too remained in India. Sanjiv has been setting up and running factories ever since. One of the happiest moments of his life came in 1986, when with the press of a button he started a ₹100 crore polyester fibre brownfield factory on the Thane–Belapur Road, Maharashtra. He had set up the factory from scratch. One of his customers was Fabina Textiles, a well-known brand of men's shirts in the 1970s and 80s. Fabina even offered him a modelling assignment for their readymade shirts. Since his company's policy would not allow him to get paid for modelling, he was happy to get a few free shirts as compensation.

Sanjiv had come on board the task force with the clear point of view that it would be frustrating for 'an enthusiastic but non-connected company like Nocca to try to be a high-quality manufacturer on its own'. In 2002, Sanjiv who was the Managing Director of Baxter India at the time, had successfully pitched a ₹38 crore factory[1] at the Industrial Model Township (IMT) in Manesar, near Gurgaon, to his US board. But despite this success, Sanjiv remained disillusioned about world-class manufacturing in India. Two years before this, in the year 2000, he had been trying to set up a small 13,000 square-foot facility near Peera Garhi Chowk in West Delhi as a warehouse-cum-office to ensure there were no 'stock outs' of critical life-saving devices. But it took him and his team four months just to get an electricity connection from what was then a government-owned utility. As always, someone in the electricity board wanted to get paid on the side, which Sanjiv refused to comply with. After writing letters relentlessly to then Chief Minister Sheila Dikshit, someone in her office intervened to get this done. Twenty years later, Sanjiv finds that very little has changed on the ground. This is why, he insists, companies like Nocca should license out manufacturing to partners like AVI Healthcare, who 'have a big role to play' in helping them expand production capacity.

On the other hand, Chirag had been doing the rounds of startup events and observing Indian medtech innovations for several years. He had seen several innovative products, but he had also observed that most had disappeared within two to three years. He had concluded that most startups had failed to effectively convert their innovation into a 'manufacturable' product. He was convinced that SMEs like AVI Healthcare could take these innovations to the market using their own manufacturing capacity and sales networks.

As luck would have it, Chirag was on one of the many ventilator-related WhatsApp groups that came up during the pandemic, some created by medtech companies to coordinate with each other, and some others for interactions with government officials. Amitabha met him in one of these groups and introduced him to the task force in early April. Sanjiv, assisted by Abhijit Sathe from SIIC, IIT Kanpur, interviewed Chirag over a call on 14 April, and instantly liked him. He made a strong recommendation to the task force that Chirag's AVI Healthcare would be a good partner for the project. The feelings were mutual, for Chirag too developed a positive view of the product as well as the team. Soon enough, on 19 April, an MOU was signed between Nocca and AVI Healthcare.

Chirag first saw the V110, and subsequently the V310. He considered the Noccarc to be better than any Indian ventilator he had seen, and on par with most international brands. He was amazed by the fact that it was being designed in the lockdown period by a team of engineers who had never seen or worked with a medical device before.

The partnership seemed like a match made in heaven. The collaboration between a talented tech startup and an enterprising SME manufacturing and distribution partner allowed both groups to play to their strengths, leading to desirable outcomes. Chirag was all charged up with new product ideas for Nocca Robotics that could help him grow his own business. The licensing partnership also paved the way for Nocca to explore other constructive partnerships. As an aside, Chirag was also excited that even though he couldn't study at an IIT, he now worked closely with a group of ex-IIT students.

Manufacturing and/or distribution partnerships between startups and SMEs make sense because it brings benefits to both. Startups have ideas, talent, technology chops and access to funding. SMEs have grit, resilience and the ability to manage the messy issues that come with manufacturing. By using the idle capacity of SMEs, startups can be asset-light when it comes to manufacturing. Incubators, investors and governments thus need to play an active role in bringing them together.

Thanks to several Covid-19 contests launched by the Department of Science & Technology[2], and BIRAC (Biotechnology Industry Research Assistance Council)[3], as well as by private foundations like Marico[4], there has been a flurry of medtech innovations developments. But how many such companies would have the stamina to manufacture and sell on their own over a sustained period of time? What if they looked at partnerships with SMEs akin to the Nocca–AVI model?

Our experience with the Nocca–AVI partnership tells us that there are four M's that need to be addressed for a fruitful collaboration: mindset, matchmaking, money and mutual respect. Each is described in detail below.

Mindset

The startup and the SME both need to develop a belief that the partnership is mutually beneficial and vastly superior to what each can do on their own. Not every medtech SME is as open-minded and objective as Chirag is and admit that the startup may be hawking products of substandard product design and quality. Chirag says, 'Go to any medical equipment fair or exhibition, and you'll see that most products showcased as "innovations" are either ragtag products or cheap Chinese imports labelled by a local distributor.' Chirag strongly believes that Indian SMEs should be cajoled to look towards institutions like the IITs for sourcing good technologies. Likewise, Sanjiv from the task force thinks that the product inventor's mindset – to build, tinker, modify, improve – is at odds with good manufacturing practices. He has seen product designers and inventors struggle to come to terms with the rigour and discipline that is needed for repetitive, controlled and process-driven manufacturing.

Matchmaking

Startups and SMEs need to enter into a durable relationship with each other. Who can 'arrange' this marriage? Most certainly incubators and accelerators should take the lead. Just as a Pitch Day is organized for startups to do a beauty parade in front of investors, or speed dating events where they can find co-founders, similar events are required for startups to showcase their products before SMEs. The government could help here through a dynamic public repository of such innovations on the MSME portal and by creating mass awareness.

Money

This is often the biggest roadblock. The startup may feel greedy and want to keep all the manufacturing and sales margins to itself, or want an unreasonably high licensing fee. Cash-strapped SMEs may be loathe to pay more than a token licence fee. There could be differences with regards to who will bear the cost of sales promotion, doctors' education, or post-sales service. While such issues will always entail negotiations, an expert group – of inventors, SMEs, incubators, manufacturing gurus like Sanjiv, and possibly an MSME ministry representative – could make the process smoother by laying out some practices and guidelines as a starting point. Since money speaks the loudest, Chirag suggests that the government can incentivize SME manufacturers by funding licensing fees through low-cost loans or grants.

Mutual Respect

Both parties – the startup and the SME – need to recognize their limitations and respect the value the other partner brings. They will both be making compromises by giving up something – the SME by giving up control over product design, and the startup by abdicating control over manufacturing (and sometimes sales). But if both can adjust to this compromise, it can lead to a long-lasting relationship.

For example, Chirag has been comfortable ever since he first reached out to the task force, and his subsequent interactions with the Nocca team have been a good experience for him. He has gone beyond his manufacturing and sales mandate to help them overcome product challenges as well. When the founders were wondering how to address one of the missing features pointed out by government doctors at the first demo in June, Chirag realized he could help. He had a proportional valve which he had procured for his own neo-natal ventilator – this could convert low flow to high flow. This valve solved the missing feature problem in the V310. He lifted his factory shutter at 10 p.m. on the night the Nocca founders drove up from Pune to Mumbai and picked it up from the security guard at 1 a.m.

This is the stuff great partnerships are made of, and this is also the way Make in India should play out – through collaborations between bright, inventive startups and resourceful SMEs. In hindsight, we should have realized much earlier that this was more likely to succeed than a mismatched partnership with a large company, especially a PSU.

KEY TAKEAWAYS

Startups and SMEs can be a marriage made in heaven.

- India has a massive number of SMEs that know how to get things done on the ground but lack innovation and technology skills.
- Talented startups can use the manufacturing and sales networks of SMEs to get a jumpstart and stay asset light.
- Matchmakers like incubators and accelerators can bring them together.
- With the right mindset, financial model and mutual respect, it could lead to great outcomes for both.

STARTER KIT

STEP 1: Incubators, accelerators, startup events and investors should actively schedule matchmaking days between startups and SMEs. They should also actively discourage manufacturing capital expenditures in the startups' financial plans and encourage leveraging the idle capacity of SMEs.

STEP 2: At the early stage, robust handholding will be required to enable a startup–SME relationship, including a financial model, manufacturing and/or distribution agreement and resolution of issues.

STEP 3: Industry bodies like Indian Angel Network (IAN) and TiE will need to work with the government for providing financial and non-financial incentives to encourage these partnerships. Industry- and government-level initiatives will be required to build SME repositories that startups can access.

Notes

1. 'Baxter India Commissions Haryana Unit.' 14 November 2002. https://www.projectstoday.com/News/Baxter-India-commissions-Haryana-unit.
2. 'CAWACH.' ISBA. https://isba.in/cawach/.
3. 'DBT-BIRAC Call on COVID-19 Research Consortium.' http://dbtindia.gov.in/sites/default/files/uploadfiles/BIRAC.pdf.
4. '#Innovate2BeatCOVID.' Macro Innovation Foundation. https://www.maricoinnovationfoundation.org/innovate2beatcovid/.

12

Dancing with a PSU

The first five minutes of the daily task force meeting was usually some light-hearted conversation while waiting for everyone to log into Zoom. But the meeting on 11 April began with some cheerful back-patting and a short round of celebration. The reason for the celebration was a tweet by Defence Secretary Ajay Kumar that morning in which he said, 'A silver lining of #COVID2019india is the eruption in related innovation across our vibrant startup ecosystem. One such case is the devt of Rs 50k ventilator by #NoccaRobotics'.[1] This tweet was also noticed by the senior leadership of Bharat Dynamics Ltd (BDL), a defence PSU. Amitabha and IIT Kanpur's phone lines immediately started buzzing with calls from BDL.

It seemed as if the ventilator project was a top priority for BDL's senior leadership. They spent hours over many sessions looking closely at Nocca's product design and development process. Discussions quickly progressed towards signing an MOU. For the task force, this was exciting because a big manufacturer like BDL would be ideally equipped to bid for and fulfil a government contract. But the negotiations turned difficult after the BDL team insisted on an exclusivity clause, whereby only BDL would manufacture and sell the ventilators not just to the government, but to anyone willing to buy in India.

No one within the task force and Nocca was willing to agree to such a clause, as discussions with other partners, especially AVI Healthcare, were at an advanced stage. BDL's argument was hard to fathom, but reading between the lines, we could see a larger PSU unwilling to cede ground to a younger startup, or to share any of the yields with a small player like AVI.

It was amusing to witness BDL's insistence especially when it was clear they did not have any sales or service teams on the ground to service small orders across the country. The MOU discussions kept going back and forth between 18 April and 28 April. To keep things moving, we agreed that discussions around the exclusivity clause could be deferred to a later stage when the final binding contract will be taken up for discussion, and the MOU was eventually signed on 28 April.

In anticipation of this big partnership, the task force brought in Asim Thakurta as the COO of Nocca on 22 April. He was tasked with managing the relationship with BDL. A seasoned executive, Asim has spent over fifteen years in a PSU, National Thermal Power Corporation (NTPC) Limited.

Asim has fond memories of NTPC's company culture. He takes great pride in its rigorous selection process, high-quality training, its habit of working with cutting-edge technologies and a constantly evolving and growing nature. All PSUs have inherent limitations that arise out of adherence to rigid rules, lack of flexibility, veto powers for finance and legal teams, but among the ten *maharatna* PSUs[2], the strengths often outweigh these weaknesses. This is why, even twenty-five years later, Asim continues to share great camaraderie with his NTPC colleagues, past and present.

Asim came into the task force just as the MOU discussions with BDL were finally coming to an end. He soon discovered that BDL was a different kind of PSU than NTPC. NTPC was much bigger, and as a prestigious maharatna, only one of ten such Indian PSUs with revenues over ₹25,000 crore. BDL, on the other hand, is one of seventy-four 'miniratnas', an umbrella term that covers all profitable PSUs.

But the difference in culture was starker than the difference in size. Unlike at NTPC, where most managers grow in the organization after joining as trainees, Asim found that BDL managers are typically parachuted in laterally from various branches of the armed forces. This results in a slow pace of work and disjointed communications within BDL. Both Asim and the task force were immensely frustrated by this, and unfortunately we could not succeed in translating this into a manufacturing relationship.

PSUs can keep pace with innovations and remain competitive by partnering with startups, but their internal culture and other organizational constraints can often create barriers for PSUs from pursuing this path seriously.

Nonetheless, with the MOU out of the way, the two teams began to work on three fronts. Technical and manufacturing teams from BDL spent time at Nocca's Pune facility to learn about the ventilator's product design and the manufacturing process. They also looked closely at the list of input components so that BDL could place orders with the suppliers anticipating a government order. Finally, BDL began to prepare a bid for the government tender.

It was with the tender process that BDL was found most wanting. Despite being a PSU, their ability to understand and navigate the tendering process was weak. And although their outstanding engineering team had understood the product and manufacturing process well and remained on standby to make ventilators in Hyderabad, the big government order never came their way – even though they had predicted the likelihood of a big order at several meetings in which all the key members of their leadership team were present.

By late June, we realized that the situation had reached a level of no progress, which came as a big disappointment to the entire task force. The MOU remained a piece of paper that did not get converted into a full-fledged agreement, and the promising relationship fell by the wayside.

Could *we* have done things differently? A lot of soul-searching within the task force finally led to a few simple conclusions about our short-lived partnership. BDL's technical team was excellent, and their speed and dedication were phenomenal. They worked hard, appreciated our work and respected us without allowing the size differential between the companies to come into play. They were aligned to our goal of manufacturing good ventilators.

But what didn't work for us was their slow progress on the business side of things. Nothing moved fast. We also noticed that BDL had a low appetite for risk; they wanted stable, predictable outcomes, and began to panic after the first DGHS demo when the Nocca team was asked to add some additional features. We were left wondering why they had entered into the relationship with us in the first place.

But does this experience mean that startups and PSUs can never be partners?

Asim thinks the bigger PSUs – the maharatnas or even the *navratnas* (a select group of miniratnas that are rated highly based on six performance parameters; there are fourteen of them, for example, Hindustan Aeronautics) – may have been better partners for Nocca because they are forward thinking. Private sector partners can often find it hard to match the ability of larger PSUs for quicker statutory clearances, land acquisitions or government support for imports. However, he too concedes that there are few examples of a successful partnership between such PSUs and startups. The exceptions that we have seen are Indian Oil Corporation (IOCL) and Hindustan Petroleum (HPCL). Srikant had met senior managers at both these PSUs several times and had been quite impressed by their keenness to bring in new ideas across all their divisions – retail marketing, pipelines, refineries and others. HPCL's pre-seed round investment in the AI startup Tranzmeo[3], and IOCL's announcements[4] of partnerships with two companies – Pepfuels and Repos Energy – for doorstep delivery of fuels look promising.

According to Dr Leena Chatterjee, Professor of Behavioural Sciences Group, IIM-C, all PSUs cannot be tarred with the same brush. 'I have seen the good, the bad and the ugly.' She believes that the dynamism of a good PSU managing director and leadership percolates downwards since PSUs are hierarchy driven. It's therefore important to get the buy-in of the leadership, build a rapport with them, and keep them engaged for things to keep moving.[5]

Although there are few non-manufacturing and non-Indian PSUs that could be termed as global exemplars of keeping pace with the times – such as Swiss Federal Rail – it is difficult to come up with local examples. Similarly, there are few models where public sector companies have successfully partnered with the private sector to use the innovation pipeline of the latter, and then manufacture at scale. Here, Professor Gautam Ahuja, Professor of Management and Organizations at the Samuel Curtis Johnson Graduate School of Management at Cornell University, recommends the NASA model of serving as a coordinating platform and hub that forms relationships with many private sector units to achieve its goals.[6]

Journalist–analyst Shankkar Aiyar, who grew up in a township in Ambarnath (Maharashtra) that had been built around two PSUs – the Ordinance Factory and the Machine Tool Prototype Factory – has strong views on how PSUs should stay relevant in changing times. For him, the models to emulate are Singapore's state-owned enterprises, the Crown corporations of Canada and the Japanese models to propel MSMEs.[7]

So, the disappointing outcome of the Nocca–BDL partnership does not necessarily mean startups and PSUs cannot collaborate. By coming together, PSUs can provide startups with massive market access, while startups can bring new innovation practices into PSUs. But there needs to be a right mix of ingredients for this broth to work. India can forge a path into the future by creating an enabling framework that makes it easier for PSUs to take the risks inherent in working with startups – these are risks that can be rather rewarding.

KEY TAKEAWAYS

Collaboration between startups and PSUs is difficult but not impossible.

- Both can benefit through a partnership. PSUs can access an innovation pipeline, while the startups can gain market access and manufacturing capacity.
- Choosing the right PSU partner is crucial. Suitable choices are likely to be only maharatnas and navratnas, where there is committed board-level support for innovation and startup partnerships.
- A robust enabling framework – including shared objectives and timelines, senior level ownership at the PSU and a review mechanism – needs to be in place early.

STARTER KIT

STEP 1: The startup needs to spell out clear reasons why a PSU partnership is necessary. The reasons could be access to a large distribution network (for example, oil PSUs), a big sales contract (such as NTPC) or immediate manufacturing capacity (such as BEL).

STEP 2: Though general managers and senior employees at the maharatnas and navratnas are fairly competent and empowered, the startup should do some background research, and also ask searching questions about the PSU board's commitment to innovation and its past track record of working with startups. Talking to some of those startups is strongly recommended.

STEP 3: Once the startup decides to proceed with a specific PSU, it is important that the MOU commits the PSU to a specific set of deliverables and outcomes in a specific period, for example, deploying the product at an agreed number of fuel retail outlets. By no means should the startup bind itself to exclusivity clauses that prevent it from working with non-competing partners or bringing in other investors.

Notes

1. Kumar, Ajay (@drajaykumar_ias). 'A silver lining of #COVID2019india is the eruption...' Twitter, 11 April 2020. https://twitter.com/drajaykumar_ias/status/1248795585072619521.
2. 'List of Maharatna & Navratna Companies in India: 10 Maharatna & 14 Navratna.' Bankersadda, 14 October 2020. https://www.bankersadda.com/complete-list-of-maharatna-navratna-companies-in-india/.
3. Dutta, Vishal. 'Hindustan Petroleum Corporation Ltd: HPCL Invest Pre-Seed Round in Startup Tranzmeo.' The Economic Times, 26 December 2018. https://economictimes.indiatimes.com/small-biz/startups/newsbuzz/hpcl-invest-pre-seed-round-in-startup-tranzmeo/articleshow/67251790.cms?from=mdr.
4. Bhalla, Kritti. 'Indian Oil Partners with Two Startups to Start Doorstep Delivery for Fuel.' Inc42 Media, 14 March 2020. https://inc42.com/buzz/indian-oil-partners-with-two-startups-to-start-doorstep-delivery-for-fuel/.
5. Dr Leena Chatterjee's interview with the authors.
6. Professor Gautam Ahuja's interview with the authors.
7. Shankkar Aiyar's interview with the authors.

13

Licence to Build

There was feverish excitement within the task force during April–May 2020 as many prospective manufacturing partners started reaching out to us eagerly. These included large and mid-size companies from the automobile, automotive components and engineering industries, and smaller ones from medical equipment. At one stage, we had close to nine conversations going on simultaneously. Even as we were warming up to some of them during this courtship period, we had begun thinking of ways to structure the manufacturing arrangement. We all knew how global technology powerhouses had built large, profitable businesses using a licensing model. Qualcomm had clocked $5.2 billion in revenue in 2018 from patent licensing.[1] Between 1991–2015, Massachusetts Institute of Technology earned $1 billion in revenue from licensing its patents.[2] Borrowing from those trends, our natural inclination was to start thinking of ways to license out the Noccarc V310 design to interested manufacturers.

But unlike these global behemoths who make a big part of their profits from licensing their technology, Indian companies have not completely warmed up to the idea of doing so, and instead prefer to make the products themselves. This is as true of medical devices as it is for many other product categories. The IIT-K task force debated this issue: should Nocca Robotics remain an inventor and license its product design to good manufacturers, or should it become a manufacturer itself?

The medtech experts within the task force cited numerous global examples of a successful licensing partnership. Sanjay Banerjee gave the example of Materialise, a Belgian company, that came up with highly innovative instruments for advanced orthopaedic surgeries, using 3D printing, which was licensed to a number of global companies[3]. A Montreal-based company had introduced robot-assisted surgeries for orthopaedic procedures and licensed out the technology to Zimmer Biomet, which eventually acquired the company. Innovation hotspots in Cambridge, Massachusetts, Silicon Valley, Switzerland and Belgium see such models all the time. But why was it rare in India for startups to outsource their manufacturing?

Former Baxter India Managing Director Sanjiv Verma thought it had to do with the lack of respect for intellectual property (IP) in India. The product and process patent regime in India was transformed in 2005 with amendments to the Indian Patent Act, which led to a sea change in sectors like pharmaceuticals where Indian companies operate globally. The Act introduced a new patent regime aimed at protecting the IP rights of patent holders and was in fulfillment of India's commitment to the World Trade Organization.[4] The 2005 amendment defined clearly what an 'invention' is and laid out three prerequisites for 'patentability' – novelty, non-obviousness and industrial applicability.[5] But within the domestic market in India, smaller companies and inventors don't feel confident that their product innovations will be protected adequately by the legal system as they don't have the muscle to defend their IP strongly and quickly. Despite that, licensing may be a way out for startup innovations in India.

In 1987, Dr Rishikesha Krishnan, the current director at IIM Bangalore, had just returned to India after obtaining his master's degree from Stanford University. He joined his father's company which dealt in professional telecom equipment – antennas – that was required by customers like the Department of Telecom, the Indian Railways, ONGC and the Indian Army. Rishi saw that his father's company was manufacturing the antennas even though technology know-how was his company's core competence, and not manufacturing. But the only reason they decided to do so, rather than license the technology to others, was because manufacturing was the only way they could make money. Licensing the technology to other companies wouldn't allow them the same profit margins.

Government-owned C-DOT (Centre for Development of Telematics), India's shining star in the telecommunications sector during the 1980s and a company Rishi admired back then, had also faced a similar challenge. Although a private telecom manufacturing industry had grown around C-DOT's EPABX (Electronic Private Automatic Branch Exchange) and RAX (Rural Automatic Exchange) technologies, Rishi recalls the manufacturers' reluctance to invest in paying C-DOT a licence fee.[6]

AVI Healthcare, the first licensee for the V310, had not seen a similar licensing partnership in the Indian medical devices industry.[7] Nocca's licensing agreement with AVI is a simple two-part model: an upfront technology transfer fee, and a royalty on each unit of product sold. The upfront fee provides a bulk payment to the inventor for all the efforts and investments in creating the product, but it also acts as a lock-in and ensures a commitment from both parties to continue with the relationship during the initial 'honeymoon' period. Nocca Robotics had discussed similar MOU arrangements with all the other manufacturers who had shown interest. Although the MOU signed with BDL did not eventually get converted into an actual manufacturing relationship. Rakesh Bhargava, former chairman of Fresenius Kabi India, says that the very act of 'a small startup signing an MOU with a big defence PSU [was] in itself astounding'.

The Indian market is at an early crossroads with respect to licensing as a business model. The believers point to global exemplars like Qualcomm, and the non-believers worry about India's weak IP protection laws for smaller companies. The medical device realists believe that when it comes to medical devices, it may be better for the company to be in control of the entire chain end to end – from product design to manufacturing to sales and customer service. This, they believe, will keep companies close to the customers, understand their requirements and create products that they really need.

A licensing strategy requires detailed groundwork to begin with. The first step is to be clear about what parts of the value chain are to be licensed out. Will the technology offered to partners be manufactured and sold under their own brand, or will it be a joint branding (as Intel does with computer hardware manufacturers)? Who will be responsible for customer education, market development and after-sales service?

Once there is complete clarity as regards these questions, the second step is to work with a good IP lawyer to draw up a draft licensing framework and agreement even before meeting up with any potential partners. The third step is to think about the commercial model. What quantum of upfront fee and royalty would be appropriate and makes business sense for both partners? The fourth step will be to draw up a list of prospective licencees who badly need a technology or invention of this kind and also have the right capabilities, mindset and market reputation. For instance, it is important to have an ISO 13485-certified manufacturing facility for medical devices. The final step is to talk to a longlist of prospective partners, arrive at a shortlist, and enter into an agreement with one or more partners.

Nocca's licensing deal with AVI can be a trendsetter for the industry and turn into a role model for other device manufacturers to partner with research-oriented inventors.

Licensing provides invaluable cash flow to the inventor by way of upfront payments, and the importance of this as a lifeline cannot be underestimated by bootstrap firms for whom 'cash is king'.

KEY TAKEAWAYS

For inventors, licensing can be a non-messy way of seeing their dreams come true.

- Inventors like to create and build products, not necessarily get into the messy areas of manufacturing and selling.
- A detailed and thought-out licensing strategy allows inventors to focus on what they like doing best, that is, designing new products.
- Careful selection of licensing partner(s) can lead to mutually beneficial outcomes.

STARTER KIT

STEP 1: The entrepreneur(s) need to decide what their personal ambitions are, and what makes them happiest. If the dream is to build a mega-corporation that designs, manufactures and sells an array of products, then licensing is not the path to take. If, however, their comfort lies in simply being geeky and inventing new products without getting their hands dirty with manufacturing, licensing could be a good way to move forward.

STEP 2: If the founders want to license out, it would be best to draw up a robust plan with an experienced advisor and an IP lawyer. This will entail a five-part implementation: thinking through and documenting the licensing strategy; creating a draft licensing framework and agreement; simulating alternative commercial models; scanning the market for prospective licensees; and negotiating with a final shortlist of partners.

STEP 3: Based on the licensing strategy adopted, there will be a need to stay engaged with the licensee on different aspects: product quality reviews, customer education, market development, product enhancements and response to market feedback.

Notes

1. 'Qualcomm Revenue: How does Qualcomm make money?' https://dashboards.trefis.com/no-login-required/O8nxFhIf/Qualcomm-Revenue-How-does-Qualcomm-make-money-?from=forbes.
2. Cohan, Peter. 'MIT's $1.9 Trillion Money Machine.' Inc.com, 7 September 2017. https://www.inc.com/peter-cohan/mits-19-trillion-money-machine.html.
3. '3D Printing Software and Services.' Materialise. https://www.materialise.com/en.
4. Jatkar, Archana. 'The Indian Patent Amendment Act 2005 and the Novartis Case'. *Trade Law Brief*, No.3/2008. http://cuts-citee.org/pdf/TLB08-03.pdf.
5. Deb, Shraddha, and Aayush Sharma. 'Section 3(d) of Indian Patents Act 1970: Significance and Interpretation.' Lexology, 7 February 2014. https://www.lexology.com/library/detail.aspx?g=3f92413f-107c-4886-aca7-24633a341e22.
6. Dr Rishikesha Krishnan's interview with the authors.
7. Chirag Gala's interview with the authors.

14

Pennies from Heaven: How Nocca Raised ₹4.62 Crore in Four Months

One of the lesser-known events in the Mahabharata takes place when the Pandavas begin their exile in the forest. Yudishthira is gifted a divine vessel, the *akshaya patra*, by Surya, the sun god. It is a vessel capable of providing an inexhaustible supply of food.[1]

The Nocca founders did not have access to such divine intervention that allowed them to have a vault of funds they could dip into when they started working on the first prototype of the ventilator in late March 2020. When Professor Govind Rajan of University of California, Irvine, endorsed their design on 27 March, the founders were excited enough to declare, 'We have enough money to develop the first working model.' They had not thought beyond that. In their idealistic pursuit, they had believed that since they were developing a product India needed, the money could soon be found. So Amitabha asked them to remain focused on the product and put fund-raising at the top of a to-do list for himself and the IIT Kanpur incubator. The founders' belief indeed came true.

On 27 March, the *Ken*[2] wrote about the ambition and efforts of Nocca and IIT Kanpur, which brought a lot of positive visibility to the ventilator project. On 30 March, Standard Chartered Bank reached out with an offer to support the team with ₹50 lakh for the initial product R&D under its corporate social responsibility (CSR) initiative. In under a week's time, the product proof of concept, task force creation and a promise of ₹50 lakh were all in place.

The next day brought more good news. The story of India's race to develop ventilators, which centred around the Nocca ventilator, was published by the BBC.[3] Although this put a lot of pressure on the team to produce results, the coverage significantly helped the SIIC IIT Kanpur team that was working to raise funding. Amitabha wrote to Dr Neeraj Sharma, Additional Secretary, Technology Development Board, and the advisor and head of Technology Development and Transfer and NEB Division, Department of Science and Technology (DST), seeking approval to utilize ₹50 lakh from an existing DST scheme named the NIDHI-SSS, one of the many government funding schemes whose evaluation and disbursement is facilitated by the SIIC. Dr Sharma approved the request, backing up a young startup with a sense of urgency and faith.

Heavenly intervention and luck were now coming into play. Within one week of starting the project, different members of the SIIC team were approached by Ansys, a US-headquartered company that makes engineering simulation software, and ICICI Securities. Aroop Tyagi, Academic Program Manager (India & SAARC) at Ansys, convinced his company within twenty-four hours to give of ₹15 lakh to Nocca as a grant for product R&D. The same week, a master budget plan to manufacture the first 300 ventilators was ready, and some members from the task force were put on the job of raising more funds. By the end of the first week of April, Nocca had completed developing the first working prototype, raised ₹15 lakh from Ansys, and got commitments for ₹1 crore from Standard Chartered and ICICI Securities respectively.

Several government and private agencies had come together to rally behind various Covid-19 solutions and launch initiatives to support innovators. The ACT Grant, a ₹100 crore grant fund, was created by multiple venture capital firms. DST launched its CAWACH (Centre for Augmenting War with Covid-19 Health Crisis) scheme[4], and another government agency BIRAC (Biotech Industry Research Assistance Council) introduced multiple schemes. The Marico Foundation launched its grand challenge, Innovate2BeatCovid[5]. The Covid-19 Innovation Grand Challenge[6] was announced by the Millennium Alliance, a public-private partnership. There were also low-interest loan schemes from SIDBI. Some agencies like BIRAC, SIDBI Bank and ACT did not even set any closing dates for the evaluation of proposals. Often the funding agencies were evaluating and sanctioning grants on a daily basis.

We applied to every possible funding programme, and during the next two months, we were selected for funding under ACT grants, the CAWACH scheme, Infoedge's CSR scheme, the Marico Foundation's Grand Challenge, and BIRAC's Covid-19 funding scheme. While it is quite normal for private funds and corporates to mobilize funds at a quick pace, it was heartwarming to witness the government funding agencies moving at a similar pace. Everyone was adapting to the new normal in an extraordinary way.

It is often said that investors hardly care for technology and are only interested in the figures on the balance sheet. But we observed the opposite. In most cases, the evaluation committee for funding schemes comprised technical experts who grilled us on our technology and ability to scale rapidly. None cared much about the business plan. And by the end of June, we had raised an additional ₹3.47 crore, taking the total to a respectable ₹4.62 crore.

What had made this possible?

The most important reason was the agility with which corporates, banks and government funding agencies moved. While being rigorous in their evaluations, they were reasonably flexible about how the money could be utilized by the startups. They broke their conventional nine-to-five schedules and took our calls even at night. In several cases, they provided more than just financial support and stepped in to help us in other areas such as customs clearance of components. Unlike pre-Covid-19 times, when startups would be grateful to get ₹5–10 lakh as prototype funding after relentlessly working for four to five months, the pandemic led to unprecedented solutions and initiatives. The empathy shown by these funding bodies was astonishing.

Another factor behind this success was the optimistic resilience of the Nocca founders and the task force members who reached out to as many sources as possible. The task force members reviewed presentations even at midnight. As a founder, Nikhil did an impressive job of pitching the ventilator. His genuineness and sincerity were infectious, in the best way possible. It is rightly said that one has to invest one's faith and money in a dream before anyone else does, and that's what Nikhil did. He made sure the funders believed in his product and his team's capability to deliver it.

There is reason to be optimistic about the future. Even before Covid-19, CSR programmes and individual philanthropy had begun contributing towards social causes. India became the first country to legislate CSR activities and mandatorily report CSR initiatives under the new Companies Act 2013.[7] Under Section 135, CSR is applicable to companies with an annual turnover of ₹1,000 crore or more, or a net worth of ₹500 crore or higher, or a net profit of ₹5 crore and above. Funds provided to approved technology incubators within academic institutions is considered part of CSR activity. This year, not surprisingly, Covid-19 has taken up the lion's share of CSR funding for many companies.[8] A Bain report shows the robust CSR growth in recent years: 'Corporate Social Responsibility (CSR) budget outlays of the domestic corporations and contributions of corporate charitable trusts, combined, have grown at a rate of 12% between FY2014 and FY2018, and they contributed approximately INR 13,000 crore to social sector funding in FY2018.'[9]

Individual philanthropy is the dark horse, however. The same Bain report shows it has grown by 21% annually for the past five years. 'These individuals currently contribute about 60% of the total private funding, estimated at INR 43,000 crore. A significant portion of this comes from a few established figures who continue to lead individual giving, as they have in the past.'

If socially relevant startups and incubators can keep companies and affluent individuals enthused about the work they do, this could be a constant source of support, and could well be the divine intervention that startups like Nocca need.

For the task force, raising funds was probably the easiest goal to achieve, and all in all, it saw a very smooth sailing. It was also the least contentious topic of discussion considering the passionate debates and arguments we had over goals like product, sales, regulation, sourcing or manufacturing.

KEY TAKEAWAYS

Multiple sources of generous funding opened up during the Covid-19 health crisis.

- CSR initiatives, government agency grants and private philanthropy all stepped forward to support Covid-related innovations.
- Systematic efforts to identify and pursue such sources helped many innovators.
- A focused and concerted approach to tap into these opportunities is possible even during normal times because India now has a robust set of CSR, grant and philanthropic funders.

STARTER KIT (FOR FOUNDERS)

STEP 1: As compared to developed countries, early-stage angel and seed investors in India tend to be more demanding in terms of their expectations regarding the progress a startup has made. Hence, startups in sectors that have long gestation periods or are not presently 'hot' sectors should build CSR and grant funding into their business plans for the first 18–36 months.

STEP 2: One of the founders should take charge of this effort. Pitching for CSR and grant funding involves not just keeping eyes open for 'calls for entries' from across the world, but also a fair bit of documentation and pitch meetings. In many cases, being connected with good incubators can provide a real-time view of such opportunities. Engaging a consultant to help with this will be a good move too.

STEP 3: It would be best to use CSR and grant funding to invest in initial foundation-building when steady revenues are yet to be seen. Angel, seed and VC investors are often reluctant to extend support during this pre-revenue phase.

Notes

1. 'The Akshaya Patra.' Hindu Scriptures, 28 October 2014. https://www.hinduscriptures.in/vedic-lifestyle/food-and-health/food-tales-from-scriptures/the-akshaya-patra.
2. Manek, Shreedhar & Kandhari, Ruhi. 'IIT Kanpur, others race Covid clock to build ventilators for India.' *Ken*. 27 March 2020. https://the-ken.com/story/iit-kanpur-others-race-covid-19-clock-to-build-ventilators-for-india/.
3. Biswas, Soutik. 'Coronavirus: India's Race to Build a Low-Cost Ventilator to Save Covid-19 Patients.' BBC News, 31 March 2020. https://www.bbc.com/news/world-asia-india-52106565.
4. 'CAWACH.' ISBA. https://isba.in/cawach/.
5. '#Innovate2BeatCOVID. Macro Innovation Foundation. https://www.maricoinnovationfoundation.org/innovate2beatcovid/.

6. 'Millennium Alliance Covid-19 Innovation Grand Challenge Call for Applications for Grants upto INR 10 Crores.' Millennium Alliance. http://www.millenniumalliance.in/covid19.aspx.
7. 'Corporate Social Responsibility (CSR) in India.' CSR Centre of Excellence. https://csrcfe.org/about-csr-in-india-public-policy/.
8. Fernandes, Kasmin. 'Top 20 Indian Companies for CSR in 2019.' *The CSR Journal: Integral Part of the Solution*, 14 September 2020. https://thecsrjournal.in/top-indian-companies-for-csr-2019/.
9. Sheth, Arpan, Anant Bhagwati, Deval Sanghavi, and Srikrishnan Srinivasan. 'India Philanthropy Report 2019.' Bain, 7 March 2019. https://www.bain.com/insights/india-philanthropy-report-2019/.

15

Twentysomethings Take on a Padma Bhushan and a Padma Shri

While racing against time to build a top-quality ventilator and faced with ambiguity on many fronts, it was inevitable that some of the task force meetings would become stressful. Matters came to a boil on 15 May when we reached a dead end trying to source high-quality flow sensors (devices used to measure the flow rate of gases going in and out of the patient). Honeywell International Inc., the go-to global giant for sensors required in ventilators, had literally gone into a freeze mode during the lockdown, and their supplies became unavailable for us in India. And, for quality reasons, we did not want to use Chinese sensors. A week earlier, out of desperation, Tushar, the youngest task force member, had offered to make our own sensors but his design wasn't delivering the required results.

On 15 May, the debate became really animated when guru–mentor, Padma Bhushan Ajai Chowdhry, kept pushing him to try harder with his own design, but Tushar was clear it wasn't possible. Soft-spoken Tushar not only pushed back respectfully, but also pulled a rabbit out of his hat. Quietly, on his own, he had scoured the globe to identify a Swiss manufacturer – Sensirion. He got them excited about the prospect of a big order from us, procured a few samples, and then showed us at this meeting that it would work. We eventually went the whole hog with Sensirion. Tushar had made his point by not just pushing back but also by relieving Ajai's stress by finding an unexpected solution.

Tushar was not the only twentysomething doing this. Aditi Kumar had turned twenty-eight in June 2020 when the task force was in operation. With an MTech in Biological Sciences and Bioengineering, a sharp mind and great attention to detail, she was responsible for ensuring that our product development, testing and certification milestones were on track. Around May-end, we were behind our deadlines and everyone was getting very fidgety. Ajai was genuinely worried about this because all our task force efforts to fight Covid would go to waste if the ventilator wasn't ready on time. At our daily meetings, he began pushing Aditi hard to move things faster. One of the suggestions was to take the product to market as soon as our designated safety testing laboratory – Swen Konformity – had certified the product. Aditi pushed back hard, 'Our final affirmation of confidence has to come from doctors and patients. We must get our product clinically validated. Let's not skip that step.' Ajai bought into her argument, and everyone's respect for Aditi went up many notches.

Debates, arguments and conflicts between new and old and energy versus experience are universal in the startup world, as are they in the world of sports. The Indian men's cricket team have several lessons for startups about this eternal conflict. In September 2005, after serving a six-match ban for slow over rates, Indian captain Sourav Ganguly was looking forward to his return for a test match against Zimbabwe in Bulawayo.[1] But he was jolted out of his comfort zone a few evenings before the scheduled match when newly appointed coach Greg Chappell showed Ganguly his selection of the eleven players who would play the match. Some key players were missing, and Ganguly was flummoxed. He pushed back at Chappell's unilateral efforts to introduce changes, which would set the stage for a messy breakdown of relationships over the next two years.

Chappell's tenure as coach was marked by pushbacks from established players. Sachin Tendulkar has famously described Chappell as who imposed his views on the team.[2] Tendulkar himself was at the receiving end when Chappell tried to push him down the batting order, to number four, during the 2007 World Cup. Harbhajan Singh similarly said Chappell's two-year tenure was an unhappy period for Indian cricket.[3] Chappell's contract was never renewed after 2007.

The Indian cricket team's coach is a tough vocation, and not many have succeeded at it. When he was the coach Anil Kumble fell out with Virat Kohli, because the latter was upset with Kumble's strict school principal-like style.[4] On the same subject, India-A coach Rahul Dravid's view seems to be a pragmatic one: 'Coaches get sacked; the first thing you know when you stop playing and become a coach is that someday you are going to get sacked. That's the reality. Players are more powerful than coaches, we know that because we were more powerful than coaches when we played.'[5]

It's not that there were no coaches who got it right. New Zealander John Wright took over as coach of the India team in 2000 under difficult circumstances but went on – in partnership with Ganguly – to create a great team. Similarly, South African Gary Kirsten, appointed coach in 2008, arguably went on to become India's most successful coach, under whose aegis the team won the 2011 World Cup. Kirsten's formula was a simple one – stay in the background, quietly offer advice, and let the team's performance speak for itself.

While the older players have experience and wisdom, the young have immense energy, talent and new expertise. Both have to come together to make a powerful team, and this involves mutual respect and minimal hierarchy. Mentorship is often subtle and uses a light touch. The best coaches, like Wright and Kirsten, rarely issued diktats.

How can we replicate the Wright–Kirsten formula in business ventures? What kind of mentors can make startup founders successful? What is expected out of experience in teams building on new innovations? These were the questions that we as task force members asked ourselves as we built a team around expertise, experience and ability. Grey-haired gurus willingly accepted the technical expertise of a twenty-three-year-old, while the twentysomethings were glad to take advice on manufacturing, supply chain or regulations from the older members.

The Nocca founders initially came into the task force meetings without knowing how the senior task force members, most of whom they were not acquainted with, would engage with them. For example, the founders had formally known Saurabh Srivastava and Ajai Chowdhry from IAN Fund who were an investor in their company, but the visits were usually restricted to Saurabh spending thirty minutes each month with them, while the founders recall being scared of Ajai. But the task force interactions were going to be a completely different cup of tea, with intensive daily interactions. The twentysomething founders were apprehensive, especially as the two 'guru–mentors' – Saurabh and Ajai – were a Padma Shri and Padma Bhushan awardee respectively.

But the founders need not have worried. Their technical expertise was sound and evident early on during an interaction with Professor Govind Rajan, the experienced anaesthesiologist from University of California, Irvine. The two quickly earned respect within the task force for their technical judgement. Soon, the founders developed the confidence to be assertive when needed, both within the task force and outside. This rubbed off on the other younger members, especially Tushar from Nocca and Aditi from the SIIC incubator.

Such interactions ensured mutual trust and respect in the team. Mentors would share best practices from their experience for several issues. The founders would take the learnings and adapt them to their reality. Mentors learnt that they did not need to spoon-feed the younger members. Warmth and friendliness played a big role in creating the right atmosphere, which is essential for any team, but even more so in one such as ours. We looked for inspiration from across the world – Silicon Valley, corporations, startups, universities and the world of entertainment – to see how constructive and energizing face-offs across generations can lead to positive outcomes.

Sriram Sankar, a senior engineering leader in Silicon Valley and now working at Uber, says that it is important to learn from the younger generation, as his own abilities in service-oriented infrastructure, big data, machine learning, search engines and so on have benefited from constant interactions with the younger generation, who are often more connected with newer trends.[6] Similarly, New York-based President and CEO of Genpact Tiger Tyagarajan sets up calls with younger people who can teach him to navigate AI and digital technologies.[7] Shreyasi Singh, CEO of EdTech startup Harappa Education, actively reaches out to three colleagues who are more than a decade younger. She describes one of them as her 'conscience keeper', while the other two who run the company's engaging podcast series 'have earned the right to say anything they like'.[8] She was once told, 'You laugh too loudly during podcast interviews.'

University classrooms across the world now thrive on such two-way engagements, and this was made especially evident during the pandemic. Ashoka University founder Dr Pramath Raj Sinha pushed for the institution to go online, even beyond the regular online classes. Thus was born the 'Beyond the Classroom' series, where twelve-hour-long lectures were offered for free to the world. To get this off the ground, he pulled in four recent alums, all in their twenties. This team had a disagreement with Pramath about the choice of technology – EdX or Google Classroom. They overcame his objections and made a compelling case for Google Classroom. Looking back now, Pramath admits it was the right decision: 'They hit it out of the park!'[9]

In older Indian universities, which largely remain steeped in hierarchy and formality, 'students expect the professor has the truth, and their job is to absorb the truth,' says Dr Rishikesha Krishnan, Director, IIM Bangalore.[10] Dr Leena Chatterjee at IIM-C is an exception. Srikant has known her for thirty-five years and seen her transition from the 'guru' approach to teaching in her early years to now seeing her students as equal partners in the learning process.

The movie industry, especially cinematography, is an interesting place to look for such engagement between different generations. The best cinematographers are usually older. The top five Hollywood cinematographers arguably are Roger Deakins (seventy-one), Caleb Deschanel (seventy-six), Rodrigo Prieto (fifty-five), Robert Richardson (sixty-five), Emmanuel Lubezki (fifty-six). Often the seventy-year-old is a lover of cinematography, stays abreast of new stuff, and has a thing or two to teach a younger person. Expertise is what is finally respected, says Bollywood producer–director Imtiaz Ali.[11]

We have spelt out a five-letter-mnemonic 'CDEFG' that can foster a collaborative environment between the older and the younger generations within a team.

1) Constant curiosity
2) Dissent inside a hierarchy
3) Expertise matters
4) Fostering a culture where respect is earned, not bestowed
5) Good social underpinnings

Curiosity is one of the biggest values cherished at Tiger Tyagarajan's Genpact. Tiger constantly tells his younger colleagues, 'I want to learn from you.' Similarly, by being curious rather than defensive, Dr Gita Johar, Meyer Feldberg Professor of Business and Vice Dean for Diversity, Equity and Inclusion at Columbia Business School, facilitates inter-generational interactions at the university.[12] Dr Leena Chatterjee acknowledges that curiosity allows her to be seen as someone who is not the only source of knowledge, and her students therefore open up and share their opinions freely.[13]

Similarly, Dr Pramath Raj Sinha learnt early on at McKinsey that an explicit company value – 'You have an obligation to dissent' – could be overlaid on the structure and hierarchy of even a large, global organization. Hierarchy may be required to get things done, but one should not fear speaking up. Chicago-based business advisor Rishad Tobaccowala hires the best young experts in newly specialized areas and provides air cover in areas he's good at – strategy, managing conflict and dealing with senior decision-makers.[14]

Dr Vijay Kumar, Dean of Engineering, University of Pennsylvania, recommends creating a culture where respect is earned, not bestowed.[15] Few simple ways of achieving this are addressing each other by first names; no private offices; same-sized desks for everyone (the CEO and the CFO can have higher priority access to conference rooms for meetings); asking everyone's opinion on important decisions; and having lunch together.

Experienced Silicon Valley techie Sriram Sankar looks for ways to bridge the disconnect in social activities between his generation and the younger generation by finding occasions to have coffee or dinner together. Good social engagement can smoothen out difficult professional interactions.

Used well, these practices create happy, productive teams where the old and young both learn from each other. Such camaraderie and exchange of ideas will certainly lead to great results.

KEY TAKEAWAYS

The old and the young can come together to make a powerful team, but it has to be founded on mutual respect.

- The old have experience and wisdom, and the youth have energy, talent and new-age expertise.
- Constructive, energizing face-offs across generations lead to positive outcomes. Subtle and 'light touch' mentoring works, not diktats.
- Five best practices that create an energizing environment: constant curiosity, dissent inside a hierarchy, expertise, earning respect, and good social underpinnings.

STARTER KIT

STEP 1: Find mentors who have the expertise but are known to be non-hierarchical and prescriptive in their interactions with younger team members. Likewise, mentors should evaluate whether the younger founders are amenable to mentoring.

STEP 2: This may not be possible in a crisis, but during normal times, a thirty- to sixty-day 'courtship period' between mentors and founders is strongly recommended. This allows both parties to gauge whether the relationship will lend itself to the five best practices outlined in this chapter.

STEP 3: Once a mentor settles down in a comfortable and mutually beneficial relationship, they would be able to refer other mentors as and when required for specific areas of expertise.

Notes

1. 'Sourav Ganguly Makes Fresh Revelations on Infamous Greg Chappell Saga.' *Hindustan Times*, 25 January 2018. https://www.hindustantimes.com/cricket/sourav-ganguly-makes-fresh-revelations-on-infamous-greg-chappell-saga/story-7Buc5pYezaarbqHbNOhwhN.html.
2. Krishnaswamy, Karthik. 'Was Greg Chappell Really a Terrible Coach of India?' ESPNcricinfo, 28 May 2020. https://www.

espncricinfo.com/story/_/id/28967400/was-greg-chappell-really-terrible-coach-india.

3. 'Chappell Was a Man with Double Face, Says Harbhajan.' *India Today*, 5 November 2014. https://www.indiatoday.in/sports/story/sachin-tendulkar-greg-chappell-harbhajan-singh-playing-it-my-way-225856-2014-11-04.
4. '"Partnership Was Untenable," Reveals Kumble After Stepping Down.' *Quint*, 21 June 2017. https://www.thequint.com/sports/cricket/anil-kumble-resignation-letter.
5. 'Rahul Dravid Condemns Manner of Anil Kumble Exit, Cringes on Some Virat Kohli Remarks.' *Deccan Chronicle*, 31 October 2017. https://www.deccanchronicle.com/sports/cricket/311017/rahul-dravid-condemns-coach-anil-kumble-sacking-cringes-on-some-virat-kohli-remarks.html.
6. Sriram Sankar's interview with the authors.
7. Tiger Tyagrajan's interview with the authors.
8. Shreyasi Singh's interview with the authors.
9. Dr Pramath Raj Sinha's interview with the authors.
10. Dr Rishikesha Krishnan's interview with the authors.
11. Director Imtiaz Ali's interview with the authors.
12. Dr Gita V. Johar's interview with the authors.
13. Dr Leena Chatterjee's interview with the authors.
14. Rishad Tobaçcowala's interview with the authors.
15. Dr Vijay Kumar's interview with the authors.

16

The Power of Osmosis

Pint-sized Aditi Kumar had spent three years as a Program Manager at IIT Kanpur's incubator (SIIC), after completing her master's in Biological Sciences and Bioengineering from the institution. When SIIC lent her to the task force, she became one of our most relentless warriors at the frontlines of the many battles fought by the task force to get the ventilator ready at express speed. One such battle was to get clear feedback from top-notch medical experts in the fields of critical care and anaesthesiology about their expectations from ICU ventilators. She was in touch with experts like Dr Prachee Sathe of Ruby Hall Clinic, Pune and Dr Rangraj Setlur of the Armed Forces Medical College, also in Pune.

In May 2020, when she was totally immersed in this work, Aditi was suddenly faced with something totally unexpected and disconcerting. An unknown person called her one day claiming to be referred by Dr Setlur and tried to engage Aditi in a conversation. Wary that this could be a competitor, Aditi kept the conversation superficial, but he kept texting her every few days. At a bit of a loss as to how to handle this situation, Aditi turned to medtech mentor Sanjay Banerjee for guidance. Sanjay had very simple advice for her, 'The next time this person calls or texts you, ask him to send an email.' She did that and the calls and messages stopped immediately.

Aditi draws a mythological analogy to describe the osmosis that was underway within the task force. 'Working with the task force was like tapping [into] a mine of knowledge. The daily two-hour calls always reminded me of the Mahabharata when Lord Krishna taught the meaning of life to Arjuna.' In Aditi's case, the source of wisdom was very often Sanjay Banerjee, and sometimes others too. When she needed help with convincing Nocca team members Harshit and Tushar about the number of certification tests required for the ventilator, she again turned to Sanjay. 'I would speak my mind openly with Sanjay, without any sugar-coating,' says Aditi.

Intense discussions with Sanjay and Rakesh Bhargava helped her learn how to do pricing for a medical device. Sanjay's spreadsheet template for pricing taught her how to do this in a structured manner, and she understood the impact of warranty policies on pricing, thanks to Rakesh's deep industry experience. One day, when she was walking Sanjiv Verma through the product development strategy, she learnt something very simple yet significant from him. Sanjiv noticed that she was updating the same document without assigning a different name or date to it. This is when she learnt the importance of 'version control', the system of recording changes to a document over a period of time.

Whether in a unique group, like the ventilator consortium, or in sports like cricket during the IPL, or while making a movie, when a diverse group of motivated experts comes together, there is a huge amount of conscious and subconscious learning from each other. Team members listen carefully, observe and work together, and absorb ideas like a sponge. When the team gets disbanded, individuals go back to their respective lives, but apply the learnings across the board. Visible improvement can then be seen in the overall quality of work.

When England lifted the ICC World Cup 2019 after a most thrilling final against New Zealand, the cup finally came home to the cradle of cricket forty-four years after its inception. It was a dramatic turnaround from the 2015 edition, when they had crashed out at group stage after losing to Bangladesh. At the time, they were said to be an old-fashioned team that hadn't adopted new cricketing tactics that had come in the wake of the T20 revolution.[1] England introspected and realized that their way of playing one-day cricket was extinct, while the rest of the cricketing world had moved ahead.[2] They now approached their game with fearlessness[3], and the result was the 2019 victory.

Former England captain Nasser Hussain believes that playing in the IPL helped English cricketers learn how to play under pressure.[4] There was no better example than Ben Stokes, the man of the match in the 2019 finals. Cricket commentator and journalist Harsha Bhogle described the IPL as the 'Davos or Woodstock of cricket' where the opportunity to learn through osmosis is huge.[5] There are life lessons galore in the IPL. Australian batsman David Warner credits his rise as a destructive test cricket player to the tips he received from Indian batsman Virender Sehwag when the two played for the Delhi Daredevils team.[6]

Similarly, Bollywood director Imtiaz Ali told us about the film industry, where people come together for periods lasting six months to two years to make a movie. Assistant directors, cinematographers, production designers, editors and many other film professionals bring together their vast and diverse experiences to contribute ideas that lead to a collective thrill, a better film and all-round learning.[7]

Osmosis is to gradually or unconsciously assimilate ideas and knowledge from each other. At the task force, however, this process happened much faster – not gradually or slowly – because of the pressures we worked under, but osmosis could be seen at work all around us. If we were to surmise what every member learnt over the ninety days of the task force, they would be:

1) Simple technologies can manage complex projects
2) The art of strategic influencing
3) The power of implicit trust
4) Making close friends without meeting them physically
5) Animated GIFs are fun

Widely available technology – Zoom, WhatsApp, phones and email – were all that we required to keep the moving parts of the task force together. Using these technologies and applications, we moved from the concept to the finished product without using an enterprise resource planning (ERP) system or sophisticated project management tools. Except for the founders flying in twice from Pune to Delhi to show a demo to the government's approval committee, members took no other flights and left barely any carbon footprint.

We also needed to learn the art of strategic influencing, that is, to be able to persuade the government-appointed DGHS committee that we had a good product; to get influential doctors excited about our indigenous ventilator; to get several small and big manufacturing partners to want to work with us; to have component suppliers ready to supply to us even when availability was scarce; to have senior bureaucrats willing to help us cut through logistics bottlenecks; and for influential print, television and online media to cover our progress. Strategic engagement with such a diverse and disparate set of stakeholders was an art many task force members had to learn for the first time.

For Srikant, it was eye-opening to see how Rakesh reached out to the best ICU heads across the country to get their endorsement for the product. Or to see how Ajai, Saurabh and Pavan identified the key members of the government appointed DGHS committee so as to try and make a strong case for our ventilator. For all his years of business experience, Srikant has never engaged deeply with the government, so he walked away thrilled with these new insights.

The task force also needed to learn the power of implicit trust and believe that others would deliver what they needed to. There was no time to second-guess expertise or intent; rather, it was assumed by all members that things would get done. If help was required, it was sought, and others would readily step in. Trust was important here, especially as we were also making friends within the task force without ever meeting each other physically. But by the time the task force was disbanded on 1 July, it felt like we were a fellowship that had come together on a quest. On this journey, older members learnt from the younger ones about the power of animated GIFs to lighten the mood every time a crisis was overcome, or a milestone crossed.

For the founders and younger task force members, the ninety days felt like an accelerated three-month MBA with five courses:

1) Attitude 101: abolishing the word 'No' from their vocabularies; learning from setbacks and moving ahead calmly; and living with ambiguity
2) Problem Solving 101: going beyond the obvious
3) Behavioural Science 101: how to be a great listener; how to delegate with confidence; how to collaborate and ask for help
4) Marketing 101: the art and science of engaging customers and media; demand generation; building an aggressive sales pipeline; and basics of pricing
5) Operations 101: project management

They hadn't expected the intensity of mentoring within the task force, and the big lessons were about learning soft skills like developing the right attitude or dealing with high levels of ambiguity. We were surrounded by ambiguity on all fronts – with respect to what the government expected us to manufacture; how much demand to expect; and whether the components that went inside the ventilator would even be available. Coping with such uncertainty while moving ahead without saying 'no' to any course of action was the only way forward. When faced with setbacks show true grit and resilience, as they did when the DGHS committee sent back the team in early June to fix missing features, and still got the ventilator approved by 19 June.

Soft skills are important life lessons for anybody in any sphere of life. But equally important are the hard skills too. Younger team members learnt how to ideate, forecast and think in advance to have a Plan B ready if something went awry.

Every discussion with guru–mentor Ajai Chowdhry was a sales masterclass. The founders learnt not to take sales forecasts at face value. Ajai ingrained in them the need to look at each sales prospect closely and ask hard questions about the real seriousness of this opportunity. He would not accept vague answers that did not provide a granular view. The concept of a 'sales funnel' came alive in their minds and was hard-coded into everyone's minds after these lessons. Likewise, Ajai coached the founders when they had to be on a television interview, and Srikant taught them how to run a sales demo.

When he heard about the ventilator project, filmmaker Imtiaz Ali saw parallels with his own work. 'In filmmaking, every film and every shot is innately unique. It's true for the ventilator project as well. The questions and challenges may be different from what team members have done before, but their experience helps them think laterally.'

Dramatic words indeed, but entirely true when a team with diverse skill sets comes together. And especially so, when the senior leaders roll up their sleeves and show the way.

KEY TAKEAWAYS

When people come together as a team, they learn from each other through osmosis.

- Team members learn from each other in surprising and unexpected ways when you bring them together for a sustained period of intense interactions.
- Some of this learning helps them do a better job of the immediate task at hand, while they take back a lot more as life lessons that help them over a longer period.
- This kind of osmosis works in every sphere – be it business or education or sports or entertainment.

STARTER KIT (FOR TEAMS AND TEAM LEADERS)

STEP 1: When you bring a team of diverse people together, besides the formal full-quorum meeting sessions, provide forums and opportunities for smaller groups to work together. While some of the osmosis-based learning happens through listening and observing others during the formal sessions, a lot more happens through active interactions in the smaller forums.

STEP 2: Ensure that, in the smaller groups, team members from different backgrounds get to mingle. For example, salespeople with non-sales, or those from one geographical region with those from other regions.

STEP 3: In case of virtual or online meetings, use focused WhatsApp groups or Zoom Breakout rooms for these smaller group interactions. When the world gets back to regular face-to-face meetings, it will be easy to use separate round tables or meeting rooms.

STEP 4: Besides formal meetings, make sure that there is plenty of time left for informal interactions among the members. When people let their hair down, they are likely to be more open with ideas.

Notes

1. Miller, Peter. 'England's ODI Turnaround after 2015 World Cup Fiasco Is Remarkable, but Bigger Challenges Await.' *Firstpost*, 5 September 2016. https://www.firstpost.com/sports/englands-odi-turnaround-after-2015-world-cup-fiasco-is-remarkable-but-bigger-challenges-await-2990548.html.
2. Shemlit, Stephan. 'How England's One-day Fortunes Have Been Transformed Since 2015 World Cup.' BBC News, 8 September 2016. https://www.bbc.com/sport/cricket/37298858.
3. Srihari. 'Eoin Morgan Credits 2015 World Cup for England's ODI Turnaround.' Sportskeeda, 18 December 2018. https://www.sportskeeda.com/cricket/exclusive-interview-eoin-morgan-credits-2015-world-cup-england-odi-turnaround.
4. 'Hussain credits IPL for Ben Stokes' World Cup Final, Headingley Heroics.' *Wisden India*, 13 May 2020. https:/wisden.com/stories/hussain-credits-ipl-for-ben-stokes-world-cup-final-headingley-heroics.
5. Harsha Bhogle's interview with the authors.
6. 'How Virender Sehwag Helped David Warner Become a Better Test Player.' *The Free Press Journal*. [Updated on] 1 December 2019. https://www.freepressjournal.in/sports/cricket/how-virender-sehwag-helped-david-warner-become-a-better-test-player.
7. Imtiaz Ali's interview with the authors.

17

Leading from the Front

As a small team working at breakneck speed for ninety days, we were managing many things simultaneously. The Nocca founders, Aditi and Sanjay focused on product design, Rahul and Rajesh on the supply chain, Sanjiv on manufacturing, Pavan on branding, while we were troubleshooting all around.

While chasing multiple deadlines on many different fronts, the task force once completely forgot about an upcoming meeting with The Millennium Alliance[1] (a global consortium that supports social enterprises in India) to pitch for grant funding. The meeting was scheduled on 2 June, and so when Ajai Chowdhry asked an innocuous question about this on 31 May, all hell broke loose. Since funding initiatives were part of Aditi's mandate, she scrambled to put the pitch slide deck together.

On the night of 1 June, she ran the pitch deck past guru–mentor Saurabh Srivastava who immediately realized that there were many gaps that remained. He provided some prompt guidance to Aditi and offered to review it again once she had fixed those gaps. It took her several hours to get this done. She finally finished her work by 3.30 a.m. on 2 June and mailed the deck to Saurabh. He was up early in the morning and had responded by 6.30 a.m. with very useful comments on specific slides relating to a few topics, for example, the impact of the Nocca innovation on the bottom of the pyramid population, project sustainability and plans for global marketing. Thanks to Saurabh's active interventions, the final presentation deck was ready and in good shape for the 2 p.m. meeting that day.

Saurabh's in-depth involvement with most issues and his willingness to roll up his sleeves and dive into solving problems was fascinating to watch especially given his pedigree and stature in the startup community. Nocca's Tushar was to witness this first-hand a few weeks later when he came to Delhi for the DGHS demo on 19 June and stayed on to visit prominent hospitals after the DGHS approval. Saurabh immediately set up ventilator demos with three top hospitals in Gurgaon – Medanta, Artemis and Fortis. Not just that, he got involved in deep discussions with Tushar about the logistics of running these demos.

Tushar had arrived in Delhi NCR with two ventilator units with the intent of doing the demos on test lungs and not live patients. But on 22 June, the doctor at the first hospital he went to – Medanta – insisted on trying the product on a live patient. Saurabh realized that any doctor worth his salt would not be satisfied with a test lung demo, and he anticipated a similar situation at the other two hospitals. But this posed a logistics challenge because once a machine was used on a live Covid-infected patient, it would not be ready to be used immediately again on another patient. Saurabh again swung into action to do a few hours of research on disinfection and autoclaving protocols and brainstormed these ideas with Tushar. Not wanting to take any chances, they also got a new machine flown in from Pune, which arrived on time for successful demos at the next two hospitals where the experts approved them.

Leading from the front by example is often the best way to motivate team members into action. It is almost always more enduring and impactful than leading by diktat. The more seasoned experts in the task force followed this principle, rolled up their sleeves to get things done. When the team needed the best critical care physician in Pune and Gurgaon to review the V310, Rakesh Bhargava and Sanjay Banerjee arranged it. When assistance was required from the government to import an urgent consignment of components from Singapore or China, Saurabh Srivastava or Padmaja Ruparel would take charge. If the team needed help moving people or equipment from one state to another during the lockdown, Ajai Chowdhry would navigate through state authorities to make it happen. Similarly, Pavan Choudary would be the go-to person for any regulatory or policy issues. The mentors were getting their hands dirty instead of merely giving advice.

In 2019, director Imtiaz Ali arrived in Chitkul, a small Himalayan village in Himachal Pradesh, to shoot for his film *Love Aaj Kal.* [2] At 11,319 feet, with the Baspa river flowing next to it, Chitkul has stunning beauty and is said to have the cleanest air in India.[3]

On one particular day, the film crew was to take a shot by the river. The location had been carefully chosen. As the equipment was being set up, Imtiaz looked longingly at an island, wondering if they could shoot from it. But there seemed to be no way of getting to the island. While the cameraman shook his head, Imtiaz started crossing over in waist-deep water. The cameraman, who knew Imtiaz well, understood the director wouldn't take no for an answer. So, he put boulders in the river, shallow as it was, and started to follow him. Everyone followed suit, placing boulders in the water and walking across. There was rain on the horizon, but no one cared and they managed to get the shot just before it began to pour.

'Two hours to get there, shoot for thirty minutes, and an hour to come back. After that, it started pouring,' Imtiaz recalls. Talking to him, one understands that his strongest memories from his career thus far are incidents such as these – where collective endeavours, often led by him, would show the way forward, with others pitching in with their support.

But we also realized that when several members begin to lead by example, it also has the potential to cause chaos in the task force. Rakesh Bhargava joined the task force about two weeks later than others and was initially unnerved by the free-flowing and somewhat chaotic nature of discussions during the daily noon calls. After spending twenty-two years in a German company, he was used to a structured environment. But the task force meetings were happening in a fast-paced, volatile environment, and it was impossible to make them more structured. He could also see the two authors bringing in some structure as project leads, and he concluded that the 'meetings were efficient, although not very structured'.

Sanjiv Verma, who also joined a few weeks later than others, had similar queries about whether a non-hierarchical work group would be effective in a hierarchal society like India. He concluded the task force worked because the two authors were accepted as project leads, given their past experience and track record at the IIT Kanpur incubator.

According to Dr Leena Chatterjee, it is difficult for a group to remain rudderless, so even if a leader is not formally appointed, one will often emerge out of most groups.[4] The informal leadership often emerges as a consequence of those who take the lead or initiative. An important condition for the acceptance of such informal leaders is their credibility within the group, which comes from expertise, trustworthiness and ethical behaviour.

Dr Gautam Ahuja is Professor of Management and Organizations at the Samuel Curtis Johnson Graduate School of Management at Cornell University, as well as Editor-in-Chief of *Organization Science*, one of the premier journals in the field. He knows of companies that have experimented with different organizational structures like boss-less firms. However, they have largely been limited to a few contexts and industries. In rare examples like the task force, he saw other kinds of arrangements, such as rotating leadership or even polyarchy (voting by all equals), emerge. But, overall, he sees hierarchy – whether mutually agreed or externally decided – becoming a staple of all groups.[5]

A fluid structure worked for the task force, with everyone leading by example. There was a complete absence of hierarchy, with the exception of some subtle nudging by the authors in a few instances. But if a similar task force is to run for a longer duration, or if a similar business acceleration model is applied to other startups, an alternative structure with some hierarchy might be required.

The ninety-day task force interactions with all the vigorous debates, mutual learning and active leadership by the seniors had, however, served the Nocca founders well. They had not only succeeded in laying a foundation for India's domestic market, but also started thinking about global markets and their own dreams of building a global product company.

KEY TAKEAWAYS

Lead by example, not diktat.

- In fast-paced, collaborative work environments, everyone needs to roll up their sleeves and lead the way in their respective areas of expertise.
- Even where formal hierarchy and structures may not be prescribed rigidly, some kind of light-touch leadership becomes necessary for ensuring good outcomes.
- Such leadership can either be expertise-based, task-based or rotational.

STARTER KIT

STEP 1: When a task force is formed, early members should lay down the rules of engagement that cover broad principles of leadership. Who, individually or in groups, will take responsibility for overall direction and the roadmap, for specific kinds of tasks or initiatives, or for periodic meetings and interactions?

STEP 2: Every time new team members come on board, they will have to be aligned to these broad principles.

STEP 3: When sufficient progress has been made, the principles of leadership can be reviewed and modified to accommodate future plans as well as the expertise and roles of new members who may have joined the team.

Notes

1. 'About Us.' Millennium Alliance. http://www.millenniumalliance.in/about_us.aspx.
2. Imtiaz Ali's interview with the authors.
3. Shenoy, Sanjana. 'This Charming Village in Himachal Pradesh Is a *Love Aaj Kal* Discovery.' *Curly Tales* (blog), 14 February 2020. https://curlytales.com/this-charming-village-in-himachal-pradesh-is-a-love-aaj-kal-discovery/.
4. Dr Leena Chatterjee's interview with the authors.
5. Dr Gautam Ahuja's interview with the authors.

BIG HOPES FOR THE FUTURE

18

Best for India, Best for the World

In the early stages of the pandemic, the world was in a state of uncertainty and panic. Without any experience in dealing with such a once-in-a-century crisis, citizens and governments everywhere were shooting in the dark. One such announcement came on 24 March, the very first day of Lockdown 1.0, when the Ministry of Commerce banned the export of ventilators and other ICU equipment.[1] This was in anticipation of a shortage in India because the pandemic was expected to grow rapidly. The export ban was not really playing on our minds at that stage because we were totally focused on first building a ventilator for India's immediate needs first. We wanted to build something very good for India.

But each member of our task force was committed to the vision of building a world-class product, while racing against time to meet India's needs. The ventilator needed to be robust and affordable for India, while eventually being ready to compete in global markets. No compromises could be afforded in this endeavour. Every essential feature and specification spelt out by the Ministry of Health and Family Welfare was built into the product and tested. Even those features listed as 'desirable' were incorporated, yet the Nocca team was aware of a few gaps.

Ventilators designed by reputed global companies have, over time, developed more refined firmware, the software program or set of instructions programmed on a hardware device that provides necessary instructions on how the device communicates with other hardware. Such high-end ventilators have dedicated modes for neonatal and paediatric categories, and a greater number of patient-monitored parameters (lung resistance, work of breathing, lower inflation point, upper inflation point, among others).

To be an attractive proposition in value-conscious India, and given the time crunch, the Noccarc V310 stayed away from additional features that are non-essential but are often attractive to customers, such as hot-swappable dual batteries and HL7 protocol for communicating with other ICU devices and central monitoring systems.

However, where the Noccarc scores over other ventilators is that it is highly suitable for the Indian market, with an affordable price point and easy operating instructions while meeting Indian regulatory standards. Riding on this confidence, the founders want to take the product global by applying for a European certification.

The logical next question is: Can the Noccarc succeed in global markets?

Dr Gita V. Johar, Meyer Feldberg Professor of Business and Vice Dean for Diversity, Equity and Inclusion at Columbia Business School, has specialized in the adoption of new products. We asked her whether the constraints imposed on Indian products stop them from being innovative and best in class. It turns out Dr Johar believes that constraints are an important enabler of creativity. The constraints on inputs (for example, resources, funding, materials, consumer price sensitivity, time constraints, and so on) paved the way for creative problem-solving because we were forced to accomplish goals against all odds. When people have limited resources, they experiment and take risks. Having abundant resources can diminish creative outcomes because it breeds complacency.

On the other hand, not having too many constraints on processes in countries like India (that is, rigid team structures or rules for interactions with peers) also allows for easy knowledge-sharing and sparks spontaneous ideas. 'I think your project came together in the sweet spot of moderate input and process constraints, enabling a creative and innovative solution,' says Dr Johar.[2] She points towards products made in India and China by GE Healthcare as examples of 'innovation under constraints'. The Mac 400 ECG machine was designed specifically for India's rural markets, and so it was designed to be portable, light, battery-operated, reliable and cheap – priced at $800 compared to the normal price of $3000 for other ECG machines. Although developed for the rural Indian market, it was sold to physicians in private practices in Europe, has got FDA approval, and is now sold to rural clinics in the US.

V. Raja was President and CEO of GE Healthcare India during 2004–11, when these innovations took place. As he says, 'Clinical outcomes are the same no matter which side of the Atlantic Ocean you are on. To address the affordability issue, retain the must-have features for India and give up the nice-to-have ones. Use the same platform to add more features for the developed world where they expect it.'[3]

Total Quality Management (TQM) expert and corporate coach Anil Kumar Sharma was a witness to the culture at GE that led to such great products. TQM is a management practice focused on long-term success through customer satisfaction. Anil attributes GE's success to the Six Sigma technique that Jack Welch convinced GE managers to embrace. Design for Six Sigma (DFSS) is an important part of the Six Sigma trilogy that many companies ignore, but GE did not. Anil believes this rigorous approach to product design led to an array of great products from the company.[4]

Many Indian companies don't seem to get how important great product design is. Globetrotting entrepreneur-cum-investor

Sunil Singh, who divides his time between Palo Alto and Noida, thinks Indian companies get two things wrong when building great products. One, they assume that because they have packed in all the features, it's an exceptional product. But while a really good product design may only have limited functionality, it will do a great job of what it's meant to do and do so reliably. Two, Sunil is both amused and aghast at how Indian entrepreneurs literally declare 'mission accomplished' when they complete a proof of concept. For Sunil, it's a bit like saying, 'My child began kindergarten today and is already prepared to face the real world.'[5]

Chicago-based author, speaker and business advisor Rishad Tobaccowala grew up in Mumbai in the 1970s before moving to the US. With a father who was chairman of Voltas and a senior official in the Tata Group, Rishad was literally living in the heart of India's commercial capital. Not surprisingly, he had a ringside view of some of India's best companies and their products in that era, which made for great dinner table conversations with his dad.

By the time he got his MBA from the University of Chicago in 1982, Rishad had fallen in love with the city and made it his home. He started working with a company that eventually got acquired by the French Publicis Groupe. Until January 2020, Rishad was Strategy and Growth Officer at the group, and his job required him to be a keen observer of products, services and customer behaviour across the world markets. He is a person uniquely placed to benchmark Indian products against those from the rest of the world. In the past he had said, 'The quality Indian products in those days were in services (Air India), food (Amul), and focused niches (Hero motorbikes). The rest were pretty crappy.'[6] But things have changed. 'Indian products have caught up in many areas when it comes to utility but still fall behind in fit and finish and the final details. On the other hand, Indian services such as hotels are better than anywhere in the world except in some key Asian cities.'

The time has indeed come for 'best for India' products to become 'best for the world' as well. Although the value-conscious Indian consumer wants affordable products, such products – if designed well – can also be world-beaters. To make this happen, Indian companies need to set their sights high, then execute plans brilliantly and relentlessly. For example, as Dr Rishikesha Krishnan, Director at IIM Bangalore, says, healthcare services companies like Narayan Hrudalaya (NH) and Arvind Eyecare have earned a global reputation for excellence through diligent innovation. NH has made high-quality cardiac surgery affordable through scale by building speciality hospitals at low cost, and by partnering with local entrepreneurs for surgical consumables. Dr Krishnan admires their transparency as well. 'Both measure their performance against benchmarks (such as success rate, infection rate, and so on) rigorously and put them out in the public domain.'[7]

Dr Pramath Raj Sinha, founder of world-class institutions like the Indian School of Business (ISB) and Ashoka University, believes that Indian ventures do not start thinking world-class from day one. While all startups start small, the quality has to be world-class from the first day itself otherwise it becomes difficult to scale quality later. In his latest venture – online education company Harappa Education – Pramath and his co-founder Shreyasi Singh have focused on providing a world-class user experience even while being an early-stage company focused on India. When they take their offering overseas, they will have prepared to become serious contenders on the global stage.[8]

But realism also needs to be a part of the thinking process. We should, by all means, aim to be the best for the world, but not go overboard while thinking 'world-class'. Anand Kripalu, MD and CEO of Diageo India, told us how McDowell's No.1 became a big brand in Africa. 'The whisky is a good product, but what is important to remember is that we are not trying to compete with single malt whiskies, but with local, possibly illegal, hooch.'[9] He recalls his days at Unilever, when shampoo sales in India had boomed because of sachets and small packs. The sachet innovation from India was taken to the world. 'Not just sachets, but sachet-making machines were also exported from India. India offered these robust machines at a fraction of the price of European machines, which were fancy but their exorbitant price just did not make sense for emerging markets like Africa.'

Indian products and services have taken two paths to conquer the world. The first is by way of brands like McDowell's No.1, Bajaj motorcycles, or even shampoo sachet machines, which have brought companies success in the emerging markets of Africa or Latin America, where a reasonably good product satisfies customer needs. Others like India's IT and pharma industries have confidently taken the second path towards developed Western markets by offering great products or services that are less expensive and help customers save money.

The Nocca founders know the V310 is a product that can be taken to world markets with appropriate enhancements and certifications. They will be encouraged by the fact that many global medical equipment leaders have designed and developed global products in India, while companies from other Asian countries have successfully climbed the perception ladder in Western markets too. Experienced medtech CEO Rakesh Bhargava (ICI, Lupin, Fresenius Kabi), now an active mentor at Nocca Robotics, prescribes a simple three-part formula for being a 'best for the world' product:

Best = (1) Quality + (2) Value for money + (3) Meet local regulatory requirements

In his view, the V310 already ticks boxes 1 and 2. And while each country has its own regulatory requirements, if the V310 gets certified by the Bureau of Indian Standards (BIS) in India, the CE in Europe and the FDA in the US, the product will find universal acceptance. The success of the Indian pharma industry should inspire Nocca founders, said Rakesh, for 'one in every three pills consumed in the US is made by an Indian company. Outside of the US, the maximum number of USFDA-approved manufacturing facilities are in India.'

While Rakesh was drilling this message into the minds of Nocca founders, the government was coincidentally moving into action around the same time. The Ministry of Commerce lifted the exports ban on August 1, while laying out its own desires, 'Now with the export of ventilators having been allowed, it is hoped that domestic ventilators would be in a position to find new markets for Indian ventilators in foreign countries.'[10]

The Nocca founders have the idealism and the passion to take great Indian products to world markets, and the continued backing of a group of mentors who believe in them. As during the pandemic, this places an enormous moral obligation on the founders to make the nation proud. And they are determined to dream bigger and bolder, and to succeed in being best for the world!

KEY TAKEAWAYS

Conquering the world is possible with both good-enough products and great products.

- Building world-class products starts with the conviction that Indian companies are capable of making one. The world-class mindset needs to be achieved early, even while the company is still small.
- Working with constraints in India sparks innovation and creativity. To channelize this into building great products requires a rigorous approach to product design.
- World-class for emerging markets or for developed markets? Being clear about this has big implications for the product.

STARTER KIT

STEP 1: Ensure that the company has a world-class mindset from day one, especially with respect to product design, quality and user experience. The product must deliver reliably what it promises, and the user must have a smooth and pleasant experience. This requires a rigorous approach to product design without taking shortcuts.

STEP 2: Once a product is successfully built and deployed in the home market, its performance should be benchmarked against the best products in the world. Does your product score better on performance or user experience or price or some combination thereof? If the product delivers reasonably good performance at attractive prices, the emerging markets of Asia, Africa or Latin America may be good markets to explore. The same product may be attractive for cost-conscious customers in developed markets. But if the product delivers vastly superior performance, user experience and pricing compared to the best in the world, it is ready for mature markets like the US or Western Europe.

STEP 3: The organization now needs a can-do mindset whereby every leader and individual needs to start believing that they are torchbearers for India in this mission and have to do everything they can to succeed.

Notes

1. Patel, Anand. 'Coronavirus in India: Day after Congress Uproar, Govt Bans Export of Ventilators, Sanitizer.' *India Today*, 24 March 2020. https://www.indiatoday.in/india/story/coronavirus-in-india-government-bans-export-of-ventilators-and-sanitizer-1659203-2020-03-24.
2. Dr Gita V. Johar's interview with the authors.
3. V. Raja's interview with the authors.
4. Anil Kumar Sharma's interview with the authors.
5. Sunil Singh's interview with the authors.
6. Rishad Tobaccowala's interview with the authors.

7. Dr Rishikesha Krishnan's interview with the authors.
8. Dr Pramath Raj Sinha's interview with the authors.
9. Anand Kripalu's interview with the authors.
10. Ministry of Health and Family Welfare. 'Riding on the Heels of Falling Case Fatality Rate, the Union Government Decides to Permit Exports of Ventilators.' Press release, 1 August 2020. Press Information Bureau. https://pib.gov.in/PressReleaseIframePage.aspx?PRID=1642872.

19

Dare to Dream

Looking back at the very beginning of their ninety-day journey reminded the Nocca founders of how far they had come. On 20 March 2020, when the chief minister of Maharashtra had ordered a complete lockdown until 31 March,[1] both Nikhil and Harshit had found themselves in an immensely stressful situation. This was a few days before the rest of the country would plunge into a similar situation. Without being able to keep their solar robotics factory running, they knew they would further get pushed into a corner even as their fledgling business was trying to find its feet. Cash was running low, and they needed to go out and chase customer orders that would keep their factory running. The state government had acted proactively after being rattled by the sudden increase in Covid-19 positive cases from fifty-three to ninety-seven in barely seventy-two hours and two deaths.[2] For the Nocca founders, it seemed almost like the end of the road. At this stage, they had not given more than a cursory glance to the mail circulated by IIT Kanpur about the Covid-19 Solution Challenge launched by Prime Minister Narendra Modi on 16 March.

Even as they were contemplating this dire situation, Saurabh Srivastava's parting words at a recent monthly IAN review meeting rang in their ears, 'Keep your eyes and ears open for opportunities.' These words, said barely a few days before the pandemic broke out in India, were to become prophetic. Very soon, the ventilator project appeared on the horizon and took Nocca towards a completely new direction that has now encouraged them to dream boldly. Something they may not have dared to do if the pandemic had not appeared out of the blue.

Daring to pursue bold new dreams is often accidental rather than the result of structured planning.

Cricket commentator and journalist Harsha Bhogle describes a similar 'accident' that had led to India becoming the centre of world cricketing power. When South Africa toured India in 1991–92 to celebrate their post-Apartheid return to world cricket, they apparently asked the Board of Control for Cricket in India, 'How much do you want for TV rights?'[3] This opened India's eyes to the monetary possibilities cricket could generate. The Hero Cup in 1993 (a five-nation tournament to commemorate the Cricket Association of Bengal's diamond jubilee) led to a path-breaking court case where the Supreme Court rejected the government's monopoly on broadcasting and opened the doors for private broadcasters.[4] This, along with the onset of satellite TV that took cricket viewership to all parts of the country, better quality of TV production, and liberalization all came together more or less at the same time to create an upward spiral. Television viewership and sponsorship money now began to originate from India, and with this, the centre of world cricket shifted. When the IPL was launched in 2008, the shift became irreversible.

What will it take for Nocca to make the transition from being a promising startup that accidentally stumbled upon an opportunity to becoming serious contenders in the big leagues?

All they may need to do is to take tips from one of the illustrious alumni from IIT Kanpur, Dr Pramath Raj Sinha. He dreamt big and stewarded the founding of two outstanding institutions – the ISB and Ashoka University – in the space of thirteen years, which is no mean achievement. Pramath's journey into education was also somewhat accidental.[5] The story begins in the late 1990s, when the Indian economy was sputtering after the initial burst of liberalization. In the absence of enough business, Pramath's employer, the global consultancy firm McKinsey, had gladly seconded Pramath to help Japanese strategic management icon Kenichi Ohmae advise the Malaysian government on how to become a knowledge-led economy. One day, Pramath was asked by then McKinsey Managing Director, Rajat Gupta, if he would like to join a team that was keen to build a world-class Indian business school. Before he knew it, he became the founding dean of ISB in July 2001, leading it after two of the appointed deans withdrew at the last minute. Pramath stayed on as the dean for a full year until Vijay Mahajan arrived from the US to take over in July 2002.

Top business schools take decades, if not centuries, to build their reputation. Wharton was founded in 1881, Harvard Business School in 1908, INSEAD in 1957 and London Business School in 1964. But Pramath and the ISB backers had a bold and audacious wish: to build a reputed business school within their lifetime. Today, the ISB consistently features on the lists of the best Asian as well as global business schools.

After the success of ISB, Pramath has made a habit out of delivering on audacious visions, repeating his success with Ashoka University, founded in 2014, which is now counted among India's top liberal arts and sciences universities. Pramath is once again on his way to revolutionizing Indian online education with Harappa Education.

Can Pramath's formula for daring to dream, setting bold goals and succeeding at them be adopted, adapted and executed by Nocca and other Indian companies? And can this exercise be expedited, since India has a lot of catching up to do?

The IIT-K Ventilator Consortium had realized early on that they were onto something special. We were not just helping a startup create a ventilator that could save lives during a pandemic but were also nurturing two promising entrepreneurs who liked to dream big and had already developed a quiet belief that their remarkably innovative product skills could power their company into becoming a strong global player.

While on campus as students, Nikhil and Harshit, the Nocca founders, had brainstormed to come up with plans for vehicles for people with disabilities, including a modular ambulance. Now with a well-designed ventilator under their belt, they are beginning to dream of building a product company not constrained by sectors. 'We want to develop high-value products with deep underlying science and technology. We want to be like Siemens,' they said. They are now thinking of high-end ventilators for global markets, non-critical respiratory devices, and non-chemical energy storage (high-wattage) devices. Their investors have backed their vision and want them to focus on large, promising product categories.

As of now, the track record of the founders suggests that they can pursue this vision without the risk of failure daunting them. Will they have the persistence and determination to keep going as the stage and stakes get bigger? Here, the company could learn from others like them.

When Anand Kripalu was made the MD of Unilever East Africa in 2004, Kenya had been losing money for ten years. His boss told him, 'You'll be the last CEO before I shut it down.' That removed all fear of failure from Kripalu's mind when he went in and allowed him to turn the business around.[6]

High-performance corporate coach Anil Sharma has an observation about Indian entrepreneurs' discomfort with failure. 'In 2003, local business entrepreneurs in Pittsburgh had hosted us. Each entrepreneur spoke about their failures, and I was left wondering why no one was talking about success. I realized Americans celebrate failure because they see it as a path to success. In India, we often hold ourselves back from taking risks for fear of failure. Our education and upbringing tend to keep many of us in a narrow box.'[7]

Similarly, Viren Rasquinha, who is the CEO of Olympic Gold Quest (OGQ), an organization that has nurtured world-class athletes like Saina Nehwal, P. V. Sindhu and Mary Kom has an audacious goal for the 2028 Olympics: athletes supported by them will win ten medals! 'Sindhu was spotted by Pullela Gopichand at eleven; she came to OGQ at fourteen, and it took seven years for her to win an Olympic medal. So even stars like her find it tough to transition from junior to senior levels. There were many moments when she did not want to continue. She succeeded, but for every Sindhu, there are many others who drop out. With the right team, talent, drive, passion, determination and strategy, anything is possible.'[8]

If the Nocca founders can balance bold and inspirational goals with a dose of realism, but without dampening the spirit of audacity, they can go a long distance. Their investors at IAN Fund have set them the challenge for Nocca to aim to be a ₹1,000 crore company by 2024! Achieving ₹1,000 crore, however impressive, means more than just a mere number. It would mean that the ventilator project has successfully provided India a new post-Covid model for building new businesses: a reinvented Silicon Valley in India. It would also mean that India's science and technology institutions and its incubators have transformed themselves. And finally, it would provide a path to entrepreneurial talent in small towns across India who would see Nikhil and Harshit's journey as one worth following. So, there's a lot at stake, and we will all be rooting for Nocca's daring dreams to come true.

KEY TAKEWAYS

Dream to fly high.

- India needs its entrepreneurs to dream boldly.
- Giving up the fear of failure and being persistent are key to achieving big dreams.
- Big dreams also need an occasional reality check.

STARTER KIT

STEP 1: Bring together a small group of people who can help you think big and boldly. These could be your investors, mentors and co-founders. Outsiders will bring in a fresh perspective, as will people who have a track record of thinking audaciously. It would certainly help if these people know your domain, but this is not always necessary. Add to this list a 'facilitator' who can provoke the group to be out-of-the-box thinkers, but also bring some structure to channelize the discussions productively.

STEP 2: Once a bold and audacious vision is agreed upon, have a candid discussion about your appetite for risks, the chances of failure, and your ability to deal with them. Asking yourself two questions – 'What's the worst that can happen?' and 'Can I cope with it?' – are often sufficient to get rid of your mind's demons. Once the fears are gone, think of ways to tackle likely difficult situations with grit and resilience.

STEP 3: A reality check is essential at periodic intervals to evaluate whether your bold recipe needs course corrections. This will ensure that the brave moves you make are not unnecessarily risky and foolish. The line between 'acceptable risk' and 'foolish risk' is very thin and blurry. It would again help to bring in your original group of experts to arrive at these important judgements.

Notes

1. Deshpande, Alok. 'Uddhav Thackeray Orders Complete Lockdown till March 31.' *Hindu*, 21 March 2020. https://www.thehindu.com/news/national/other-states/uddhav-thackeray-orders-complete-lockdown-till-march-31/article31123771.ece.
2. Najmi, Quaid. 'Maharashtra Imposes "Total Lockdown" as COVID-19 Cases Reach 101.' *The Weather Channel*, 24 March 2020. https://weather.com/en-IN/india/news/news/2020-03-24-maharashtra-imposes-total-lockdown-covid-cases-reach.
3. Harsha Bhogle's interview with the authors.
4. 'By Rejecting State Monopoly on Airwaves, Supreme Court Opens Door for Private Broadcasters.' *India Today*, 15 March 1995. https://www.indiatoday.in/magazine/society-the-arts/media/story/19950315-by-rejecting-state-monopoly-on-airwaves-supreme-court-opens-door-for-private-broadcasters-806996-1995-03-15.
5. Dr Pramath Raj Sinha's interview with the authors.
6. Anand Kripalu's interview with the authors.
7. Anil Kumar Sharma's interview with the authors.
8. Viren Rasquinha's interview with the authors.

20

Silicon Valley Reinvented

This time it was an email that started it all. If the ventilator project started for Srikant with a phone call from Amitabha on 27 March, now it was an email he received from IIM Calcutta on 23 July that set him off on a new project.

The task force had been disbanded on 1 July 2020 once the Noccarc V310 had got clinical validation, and a full-time team took charge at the company. Task force members who initially showed withdrawal symptoms were getting back to their normal routines. Srikant had once again begun focusing on his own pre-Covid work portfolio – advising clients, mentoring startups and incubators and teaching as a visiting faculty member at Ashoka University. Barely three weeks later, Srikant received an email from his other alma mater IIM-C. Professor Balram Avittathur, the head of Centre for Entrepreneurship and Innovation (CEI) at IIM-C had invited him to address the incoming batch of 480 MBA students in early August.

His mind still bursting with ideas from the ventilator project, Srikant quickly mooted the idea of going beyond a mere welcome speech. He suggested creating a programme that would offer a ringside experience of entrepreneurship to a select group of these MBA students. Everyone was excited about this – Professor Balram, Professor Anju Seth (Director, IIM-C), Subhrangshu Sanyal (CEO, IIM Calcutta Innovation

Park) and Nikhil Chaitanya Madaram (President, Students Entrepreneurship Cell).

A few conversations later, this group had agreed upon a full-blown plan. The Post-Covid Venture Experience (PCVE), a six-month programme was announced by Srikant on 5 August to the incoming batch. Five promising startups from IIM Calcutta Innovation Park (IIMCIP) were selected for accelerated mentoring along the lines of the ventilator project. Each startup would be supported by a distinct task force of experts each comprising two experienced alumni mentors, one faculty member, two MBA students and one senior member from IIMCIP. The task forces would meet over Zoom every Saturday from October 2020 to March 2021 with the aim of making these five startups investor-ready.

With this, our ventilator task force model was now ready for its next phase, replication and expansion, with two significant differences and several similarities. The first difference was in the frequency of the meetings – weekly instead of daily. The other difference was the vastly expanded coverage of industry sectors – the five startups spanned healthcare, rural livelihoods, logistics, drones and 3D figurines. The main similarity between the two models was in the quality of people in each of the task force. The best mentors were brought in for each startup, and they were geographically dispersed – Kolkata, Delhi, Mumbai, Bengaluru and Singapore. The PCVE programme was formally launched on 17 October, and there are high expectations around it because – building on the experience of the ventilator project – it is a real experiment around reinventing Silicon Valley in India.

Sriram Sankar is the quintessential Silicon Valley techie. After a PhD in Computer Science from Stanford University in 1989, he worked for the great pre-internet era company Sun Microsystems before founding his own startup, Metamata. After running it for four years, he sold it in 2001 to Webgain, a BEA Systems subsidiary. Since then Sriram has worked in senior engineering roles at several other Silicon Valley companies: VMware, Google, LinkedIn, Facebook and Uber. He has seen the Valley create magic through a continuous stream of innovative products and many of those eureka moments when teams have unearthed great ideas. Sriram recalls brainwaves that arose out of free-flowing conversations at a party, or while playing a game, or just driving together somewhere, and eventually turning big.

The pandemic forced everyone in Silicon Valley to work differently through remote collaboration. Sriram finds this has compromised people's ability to be as inventive and collaborative as before. The inherent formality and preciseness of Zoom calls coupled with distractions that come from having to multitask makes the collaboration sub-optimal. The absence of spontaneous whiteboarding and water-cooler conversations impedes creativity.

Sriram has tried to improvise by physically meeting a small number of people willing to go on socially-distanced walks, which has worked for him. But he believes people will be less efficient in the current pandemic than if they were working in person. This will (at least temporarily) rob places like Silicon Valley of its advantage over other locations: 'Right now, it does not matter if one lives in Silicon Valley or Dehradun or Nigeria. All they need is a good internet connection and the willingness to adjust to the time difference.'[1]

Silicon Valley has been a unique place where top universities, global talent and capital are all concentrated within a 50 square mile area, where bold ambitions and no-holds-barred ideas have come together to create innovation and wealth. Countries like India could not match it, and cities like Kanpur and Kolkata could not even begin to dream about it. But our task force has created a new paradigm where space and time no longer posed constraints. Top universities; global talent, especially from the Indian diaspora; and capital were brought together in the virtual world. The ventilator project is thus a successful template to reinvent Silicon Valley in India and could very well be replicated for other ventures to create world-class companies.

On that note, why not rewind to how the project took shape.

During the early stages of the pandemic, the 'problem statement' ('Can any of your startups design a ventilator?') originated from the government and was broadcast widely by the SIIC incubator at IIT Kanpur to more than 140 startups. The founders from one such startup, Nocca Robotics, came up with an initial design idea. A diverse group of mentors created a task force to help improve the design and accelerate its transformation into a viable product in record time. The mentors helped bring in capital, fresh talent, advice, access to government and other experts and the ability to overcome roadblocks. The founders and mentors were supported brilliantly by the operating team at the incubator that ensured multiple workstreams stayed on course.

In this model, an Indian venture based in a non-metro city got remote access to a rich array of resources from across the world. This happened at great speed, with frugality, and resulted in high-quality outcomes, including social impact.

So, can this new paradigm reinvent the Silicon Valley model in India and for the times we live in? We spoke to several experts across the world about whether the ventilator project could be a minimum viable product (MVP) for this new paradigm.

Professor Gautam Ahuja of Samuel Curtis Johnson Graduate School of Management at Cornell University, who has done extensive research in the areas of technology, innovation and globalization, believes it is a wonderful aspiration to work on such industry–university–VC collaborations as the task force and is hopeful that the model can be scaled up.[2] He recommends a few more demonstration projects that solve some real problems and bring together the right task force as in the ventilator project to establish this model. Steady scaling up through a stream of successes is the way forward. For us, the PCVE programme at

IIM-C brings forth those next set of demonstration projects whose potential success will fuel further scaling up of the model.

Palo Alto and India-based investor Sunil Singh thinks it is not foolish to see the task force as 'Silicon Valley Reinvented'.[3] He finds this happening in some areas already. Software products are being increasingly built with globally distributed teams. But he has divergent views on what it would take to build products for the Indian market versus the ones for the global market. In the latter, he believes some of the team members must be based in locations close to key global markets so that they can build customer-centric products. For instance, if a startup wants to sell tech products in the US market, part of the team must be based there and get early customer validation.

For Yashdeep Kumar, Vice President of Global Innovation at Stryker Corporation, 'This [task force] model is the best thing that has happened.'[4] To scale this up, the key would be a deep engagement with the alumni of India's top technology institutions as well as the broader Indian diaspora. In sectors like medical devices, there may not be enough grey-haired veterans with relevant experience, so one can look at related areas like pharmaceuticals to find the right mentors.

While the task force model can be used to rapidly build products and ventures of the kind one sees in Silicon Valley, the real opportunity may lie in exploring new and additional frontiers that are unique to India and other emerging markets. There are a range of unsolved problems in agriculture, health, education, drinking water, sanitation, electricity access and livelihoods – the list is endless. One could argue that Indian startups and unicorns are already addressing these challenges – PayTM is enabling financial inclusion; Byju's is improving access to high-quality education; ReNew Power will make clean energy available to the country at large. But the truth is that India's real problems remain untouched by the startup world. The startups who are involved tend to be smaller, and the investors who back them are described as 'impact investors'.

In his book, *The Gated Republic: India's Public Policy Failures and Private Solutions*, Shankkar Aiyar describes how citizens are moving away from dependence on the government towards private providers for basic services like drinking water, dependable power supply, good primary healthcare, education and safety.[5] If the 'Silicon Valley Reinvented' model can bring together the right technology, capital and business model with a group of committed founders, mentors and champions to solve these massive problems, we can actually move the centre of gravity to India. This model can be applied in other emerging markets as well.

Indians have produced sixty-one startup unicorns, but only twenty-one are based in India. The rest are based overseas, and mostly in Silicon Valley. Facts like these, or that the CEOs of Microsoft, Google, IBM and Adobe are all of Indian origin, prompts Chicago-based advisor Rishad Tobaccowala to say, 'Silicon Valley was in India, but it migrated to the West.'[6] He believes that the stars are now aligned well enough to reverse the direction and bring a reinvented Silicon Valley into India because of three breakthroughs:

1) Cloud is the new Silicon Valley in the sky.
2) High-bandwidth (5G) communication allows people to connect with each other and the cloud.
3) Every business depends on software in some form, and so every business is a tech business.

Senior mentor to the task force Ajai Chowdhry believes we can run 'super accelerators' in India where the best global teams can be created with the power of connectivity and imparting skills across technical and business mentoring, go-to-market strategy, product development, manufacturing, after-sales service, sourcing, legal, funding, and so on. The time a product takes to reach the market can be reduced without compromises.

Logic and the rational mind strongly suggest that India has a once-in-a-lifetime opportunity to reinvent Silicon Valley. But there is a big non-rational factor at play here that may be hard to recreate in this new model. This has to do with the magic of living in Silicon Valley in the midst of a massively connected graph of people. Sunil Singh, an investor who divides his time between Palo Alto and India, described how he stumbled upon some big opportunities thanks to this magic, 'Living in the Bay Area definitely has the advantage that you are in the midst of constant and frenetic activity. Many of my Saturday mornings and evenings have been spent at what used to be called the old University Café, poring over a laptop, reviewing demos and early prototypes. There have been innumerable ideas and partnerships that have come as a direct result of these serendipitous meetings.'

Sunil remembers how he had met a really bright founder, Rajat Paharia, over a cup of coffee. 'Paharia was thinking of doing his own startup and wanted to chat about several ideas. We batted around a whole bunch of ideas, many "crazy" ones. This led to our founding of Bunchball, a "gamification platform" – sketched over a napkin in the Starbucks at Redwood Shores – where I became the founding investor and board member, and which raised several rounds of venture financing and exited in a PE transaction – and is today deployed in hundreds of corporations – and Rajat became the de facto "father of gamification".'

Besides several investing opportunities that he unearthed during such casual coffee conversations, Sunil believes he has grown personally through chance encounters with inspirational people, 'It's not just the early founders you get to meet. The power of Silicon Valley is this vast network of knowledgeable and relevant people – it's all a connected graph – and you end up traversing the graph along the edges from one node to the next, propelled by one introduction to another. I remember, in early 2005, having been invited by a friend for a breakfast meeting.

One of the people at the breakfast table was Reid Hoffman (well-known American internet entrepreneur and the co-founder of LinkedIn), and in that hour, I learnt all about Reid's thinking around what he looks for in a successful internet business – I learnt about LinkedIn (which I didn't know well at the time) and why a professional network would be successful.'

The ultimate landmark meeting for Sunil was in early 2000, where over a cup of coffee, the late Rajiv Motwani (Professor of Computer Science at Stanford University, an advisor to many startups, and a friend of Sunil) introduced him to two budding entrepreneurs who were trying to reinvent internet search. 'While I questioned them sceptically on why they were working on internet search which was already crowded with so many players (I viewed Alta Vista as the frontrunner), Rajiv and the two entrepreneurs patiently explained the uniqueness of "relevant search" and the page-rank algorithm. The two entrepreneurs were Sergey Brin and Larry Page of Google.'

Can this magic of Silicon Valley, through many planned and unplanned interactions, be recreated and reinvented in India?

If ever there were a chance to do this, it is now – especially in the post-Covid era – when a part of Silicon Valley's traditional advantage may have diminished. In this new collaborative world, India can bring together ideas, young talent, experienced mentors, and capital unhindered by their location. The Indian entrepreneurial DNA, coupled with tech breakthroughs and the world's frustration with respect to China, makes it the right time for India to dream big. Especially if this is backed strongly by our startup incubators, science and technology institutions and the government the way they did during the pandemic.

KEY TAKEAWAYS

It's time to reinvent Silicon Valley in India.

- Silicon Valley holds a unique place in the startup world, and its impact is literally magical.
- Many of Silicon Valley's big advantages have become weakened during the pandemic, and this is a real opportunity for India to create an alternative model.
- The weak physical infrastructure in most Indian cities, and especially the smaller cities, does not have to be a disadvantage any longer in an era of remote collaboration.
- By leveraging the best expertise across India and the world, Indian startups can become world-beaters, and also aim to solve some of our most pressing problems concerning agriculture, health, education, drinking water, sanitation, electricity access and livelihoods.

STARTER KIT (FOR INCUBATORS, VCs AND GOVERNMENT AGENCIES)

STEP 1 (SIX MONTHS): Replicate the 'ventilator project' model with a few more startups focused on key sectors such as medtech or edtech. All the elements from the model (for example, an expert task force; speed of execution; government support; incubator participation; focus on results) should be tested again with three to four startups. Fine-tune the model by demonstrating success over next six months.

STEP 2 (SUBSEQUENT EIGHTEEN MONTHS): Pick two to three sectors for massive scale-up of this model. These should be sectors where India faces an unsolved problem (for example, quality healthcare for the masses), where the government will commit to demand generation through policy interventions that support local innovations and manufacturing.

STEP 3 (BEYOND THE FIRST TWO YEARS): Once this model scales up in India, it would be the right time to take products and services to other emerging markets.

Notes

1. Sriram Sankar's interview with the authors.
2. Dr Gautam Ahuja's interview with the authors.
3. Sunil Singh's interview with the authors.
4. Yashdeep Kumar's interview with the authors.
5. Shankkar Aiyar's interview with the authors.
6. Rishad Tobaccowala's interview with the authors.

21

A World-beating Formula for Incubators

Back from the ventilator task force in early July, Amitabha's mind was buzzing with ideas, just like Srikant's. But he was also a worried man. He had realized that, to stay relevant and succeed in the post-Covid world, the SIIC incubator would need to transform completely. No longer could the incubator be just a platform for evaluating funding requests from startups and disbursing them on behalf of government grant-giving agencies, with some mentoring and optional infrastructure thrown in.

Always impatient for action, he began firing on all cylinders and moving forward on several fronts after a brainstorming session with the SIIC incubator team. First, having seen the talented young Nocca engineers at work in the ventilator task force, he decided to go one step further by engaging current BTech students at IIT Kanpur. To do this, he created a one-year fellowship programme where graduating students could opt for 'deferred placement' to actively pursue entrepreneurship at SIIC and come back to seek placement two years later if they wanted to. Two students have already been offered fellowships after a selection process, and they will soon begin work on developing prototypes for real market-driven problems, one of which has been identified by AVI Healthcare, the manufacturing partner of Nocca Robotics.

The second step Amitabha took was to sign partnership agreements with three well-known medical device companies – BPL Healthcare, Siemens Healthcare, and Allied Medical. These partnerships will enable SIIC to create a stronger presence in healthcare innovation by providing its startups opportunities for mentorship, market access and funding.

The final step was to extend the same approach to other sectors. He picked edtech (technology-enabled education) and fintech (technology-enabled finance) to start with. To ensure these forays were market-driven, SIIC launched the 'Hack & Reboot' event[1] in September, a national-level digital hackathon, where startups were invited to develop technology solutions for problems identified by experts from these sectors.

Covid was clearly a wake-up call that taught new skills to incubators like SIIC. The experience with the task force was a crash course for SIIC team members, and they learnt a new world-beating formula to transform the incubator itself. They also learnt other lessons by helping and observing some of their other incubated startups as well. Sandip Patil's eSpin Nanotech that produces face masks under the brand Swasa was one of them.

Sandip's success is indicative of what India's technology incubators can deliver to the country if they reorient themselves. Sandip pursued his PhD at IIT Kanpur from 2006 to 2012, translated his research topic (nano-fibre technology) into a business idea (making lab-scale machines for nano-fibre spinning), and successfully sold 215 machines to academic and research institutions in India, the Middle East and Europe. He continued to dream big by working on an industrial-scale machine to make masks that could be worn in India's polluted cities. With no capital in hand, he started this venture in 2018 with a contract manufacturer in Gujarat. And when the pandemic started to rage in March, he quickly imported a machine worth ₹2 crore to start making PM0.3 masks for virus protection.[2]

Not every aspiring entrepreneur can have a dream run of this kind. Sandip's journey became a reality because his PhD guide, Dr Ashutosh Sharma (now Secretary, DST), encouraged him to pursue his startup dream alongside his doctorate. IIT Kanpur's incubator (SIIC) showed him how to set up a company, and he had access to all the labs on campus, including the chemical engineering ones. When he wanted to import a machine that cost ₹2 crore, during the pandemic, he got help with arranging a ₹50 lakh grant, a 3,000 square-foot space and a lot of moral support. And finally, on 5 August 2020, he got another lucky break!

It was the day of the high-profile *bhoomi pooja* of the Ram mandir in Ayodhya, and Sandip's colleagues had spotted Prime Minister Narendra Modi wearing their Swasa face mask. The Swasa design was unique and distinctive, and the logo became visible when the TV cameras zoomed in on the PM.

Sandip was completely taken by surprise. The PM had worn it once in the past, while on an aerial tour of West Bengal to survey the damage caused by Cyclone Amphan in May that year. Sandip still doesn't know where the Prime Minister's Office (PMO) procured the masks from. It is possible that his Lucknow distributor Blue Heart Care had sent it to the PMO, and they may have also been sent via an IAS officer in Gujarat. Back in March, when Covid cases had started rising in Gujarat, an IAS officer had called IIT Kanpur's director to inquire about the masks being produced by an IIT-K startup. Sandip's masks were being manufactured by a third-party in Gujarat, and he had immediately provided 10,000 masks to the Gujarat government.

Did the sudden visibility help Swasa sales grow? Sandip finds it difficult to answer the question because mask sales have generally boomed. But his distributors and dealers are certainly enthused on having seen the PM wearing their mask. Forty thousand masks are now being made each day at Sandip's two factories, a number that could go up to 50,000 if needed. The

Gujarat factory, which makes PM2.5 masks, has been making them since September 2019, while the new Kanpur factory, which went live during the pandemic, produces PM0.3 masks. Swasa masks use nano-fibre technology with a special PVDF fibre as its core that is used in applications requiring the highest purity and are FFP certified. Filtering Facepieces Protect, or FFP, is a mechanical filter standard used for protective respirator masks by the European Union.[3]

The 150 technology business incubators (supported by the government's DST) and fifty bio incubators (backed by BIRAC, the semi-autonomous entity set up by the Department of Biotechnology) have done a good job of taking the message of entrepreneurship across the country to over hundred cities.[4] An objective report card would give them top grade for providing innovators with access to funding, workspace, technology advice and labs. But they haven't done as well in mentoring businesses, supporting scale-ups, making entrepreneurs investor-ready, and providing expert advice in specialized areas like structuring tech transfer arrangements, such as licensing.

What made incubators like SIIC, and several others, bloom during the pandemic was that the government began to use them as a massive communication network to urgently identify relevant innovators. The incubators are familiar with the innovators and their capabilities. The moment the specific requirements for Covid-19 became clear – ventilators, masks, face shields, PPE kits, sanitizers, and so on – the incubators swung into action to put forward their best startups. These startups, when faced with the urgency of the situation, became fearless. Dr Nikhil Agarwal, CEO of IIT Kanpur's incubator, says, 'Risk-taking ability increases significantly when you set aside calculations of risks and benefit.'[5]

Nikhil's team encouraged eleven startups to develop products and services to combat the pandemic, including a sensor-enabled sanitization tunnel, intelligent disinfection chambers, automated

UV sanitization of smart toilets, and smart bins for safe disposal. As part of the task force himself, Nikhil believes that being an underdog helped since 'nobody believed we could pull this off with people who were part-timers, but we became a formidable force coming together'.

For the regular staff of Nikhil's incubator team, the task force was an accelerated ascent from adolescence to adulthood, the best example being Rahul Patel, a talented engineer who is already working on his second startup along with working for the incubator. In his regular role at the incubator prior to the task force, he didn't feel challenged enough because he was some distance away from the actual action happening at the incubated startups. But through the task force, he became an extension of the Nocca team, and was assigned the crucial responsibility of sourcing. 'Never in my wildest dreams did I imagine managing supply chains,' he says.

A similar story was playing out at many incubators across the country. In various cases, incubators used a light touch to support self-motivated startups. For example, the Pune-based MyLab Discovery Solutions developed India's first indigenous approved RT-PCR kit as early as March.[6] When they needed help with raising funds to develop multiplexed kits that would be a cost-effective method and led to faster detections, Venture Center[7], India's largest science business incubator, stepped in to find them a CSR funding of ₹90 lakh. Venture Center also helped PadCare Labs – whose original claim to fame was 'the world's first smokeless sanitary pad disposal machine', an ultraviolet (UV) disinfection system for sanitizing sanitary pads – develop related applications for the re-use of N95 masks and an UV-based sanitization system for disinfecting surfaces and aerial contamination. Here, Venture Center's support ensured that the startup had access to labs, as well as regulatory, technical and market-related advice.[8]

Similarly, about fifteen of the sixty startups incubated at the IIMCIP came up with Covid-related products and services.

One of them, tele-radiology startup 5C Networks, saw their business decline in the first month of the lockdown until they developed a Covid-related offering. The startup's teleradiology solution scans lungs and the digitized images can be viewed remotely by doctors. Using machine learning, 5C is now able to interpret whether a person is Covid-infected along with the severity of the infection. IIMCIP estimates that, by the end of August 2020, 5C Networks was reporting over 1,000 suspected Covid-19 cases daily through their machines, with over 20,000 Covid-19 reports overall. [9]

Incubators also turned into frontline warriors during this time. Venture Center played a stellar role in making face shields available in Pune when the need was dire. 'We formed an action group for face shields in March when the Pune police requested our help,' says Dr V. Premnath, CEO of Venture Center and head of CSIR-NCL Innovations.The key challenge was in getting the right raw materials to keep the price at less than ₹25 per shield. Because of high costs, 3D printing was ruled out. So, the Pune Face Shield Action Group then made face shields with a medium-density fibreboard (MDF) frame and plastic sheets in April and May. An amount of ₹25 lakh was quickly raised through small contributions, and 1 lakh face shields were donated in April itself. By mid-May, two startups were encouraged to come together and produce face shields commercially. Their brand, Armor, is now available in the market.

Similarly, new models of collaboration began to emerge between startups, and between incubators too. Agastya Buoyant, a startup incubated at IIMCIP, collaborated with Abstract Ideas, an IIT Bombay startup, and two others, to create Arogya Kavach, which claimed to be the first anti-viral, breathable, washable and reusable PPE. These startups came together organically on their own. On the other hand, the National Science and Technology Entrepreneurship Development Board's (NSTEDB)10 CAWACH initiative brought together several leading incubators under one umbrella. Under CAWACH (Centre for Augmenting War with COVID-19 Health Crisis), which was set up at the end of March 2020 with a budget of ₹150 crore, 800 funding applications were received from innovators, which went through three levels of screening. Finally, fifty-one startups were eligible for funding by July end. In this scenario, incubators, instead of competing with each other, pulled in all their resources to turn CAWACH into a successful initiative.[11]

But not all incubators were similarly active during the lockdown. Vijaya Kumar Ivaturi, an active mentor to startups at many incubators and accelerators across the country and the author of *The Manual for Indian Startups*, found that incubators with a prior focus on biotech, medtech or healthcare could pivot their startups to Covid-related products and services, but others couldn't. Personally, he was delighted when one of the startups he has mentored, Thinkerbell Labs, which made devices to teach Braille, leveraged its core skills to design a low-cost infra-red thermometer that attaches itself to any smartphone.[12]

Dr Nikhil Agarwal dreams of replicating the Nocca model at SIIC to create more winners. His formula is to create cohort-based innovation programmes (like the famous startup accelarator Y Combinator in the US that, since its launch in 2005, has supported over 2,000 companies including well-known ones like Airbnb, Dropbox and Reddit), rather than work with individual innovators. Dr V. Premnath saw that startups had learnt that go-getters stood out, and that speed and adaptability mattered. Dr Anita Gupta, head of NSTEDB, now wants incubators to become true centres of excellence by playing proactive roles in mentoring promising startups. Inspired by CAWACH, she believes collaborative platforms will have a big role to play in the days to come.

For entrepreneurs like Sandip Patil this will be music to the ears. He came from a poor farming family in Dhule, Maharashtra. An incubator made it possible for him to become an entrepreneur, create jobs, and dream of giving back to Kanpur by creating his own incubator. With a likely revenue of ₹20 crore in Financial Year 2020–21, he is already thinking of what the not-too-distant future will look like.

India's incubators have discovered a new formula during the pandemic, and now there is hope that we can create many world-beating companies. Working in close partnership with our eminent science and technology institutions and the government, this now looks like a distinct possibility.

KEY TAKEAWAYS

The emergence of Indian incubators version 2.0.

- Over the past decade, India has seen a wide network of incubators that have kept pace with the spread of startup culture. But these incubators have had a mixed track record in terms of genuine value addition.
- The Covid-19 crisis enabled several incubators to acquire a new set of capabilities in an accelerated mode. Risk-taking, creating robust mentoring frameworks, active engagement with startups, and collaboration with other incubators are new skills they have acquired in this time.
- This new generation of incubators is now well-poised to nurture world-beating startups.

STARTER KIT (FOR INCUBATORS)

STEP 1: Spell out a clear vision and objectives for the vision through a consensus-based approach by involving your key stakeholders – your host institution or state government or business leaders in your city. Try and create a distinctive vision by focusing on the strengths and aspirations of your host institution or geographical region. For instance, if your host institution is an engineering college with strong civil engineering and architecture departments, it makes sense to align your incubator accordingly. Or, if you are based in a less-developed state, focusing on the socio-economic challenges of that state would make your incubator very relevant.

STEP 2: Look for sourcing and incubating startups that are aligned with your vision.

STEP 3: Support these startups through strong mentoring programmes and by providing access to an array of funding schemes – both government and private – and other support services.

Notes

1. 'Hackathon-TIDE.' SIIC IIT Kanpur, 10 October 2020. https://siicincubator.com/hackandreboot/.
2. Dr Sandip Patil's interview with the authors.
3. 'FFP Standards.' Wikipedia. Wikimedia Foundation, [Updated on] 3 January 2021. https://en.wikipedia.org/wiki/FFP_standards.
4. Dr Anita Gupta's interview with the authors.
5. Dr Nikhil Agarwal's interview with the authors.
6. Rajagopal, Divya. 'Pune-based Mylab Becomes First Indian Company to Get Covid-19 Test Kits Validated.' *Economic Times*, [Updated on] 24 March 2020. https://economictimes.indiatimes.com/industry/healthcare/biotech/healthcare/pune-based-mylab-becomes-first-indian-co-to-get-its-covid-19-test-kits-validated/articleshow/74785575.cms?from=mdr.
7. 'Venture Center: Technology Commercialization, Business Incubator India.' Venture Center. https://www.venturecenter.co.in/. https://www.venturecenter.co.in/.
8. Dr V. Premnath's interview with the authors.
9. Dr Subhrangshu Sanyal's interview with the authors.
10. 'Welcome to NSTEDB.' NSTEDB. http://www.nstedb.com/.
11. Dr Anita Gupta's interview with the authors.
12. Vijaya Kumar Ivaturi's interview with the authors.

22

A Strong Comeback by Science and Technology Institutions

On a normal day, the innately picturesque 1055-acre campus of IIT Kanpur is a calming antidote for busy minds hurrying towards their classes. Though a mini academic city, it does not have the noise, dust or traffic of a normal Indian city. The peace is only occasionally disturbed by the beautiful peacocks moving across the green grounds. It was even quieter in the summer of 2020 when the campus was more than half-empty with students having been sent home for the lockdown.

The campus started buzzing with a different sound on 18 June when the erstwhile Students Activity Centre ('The Old SAC') became a commercial production centre for the SWASA N-95 mask. A fully automated manufacturing facility with a daily capacity of 25,000 masks had gone live that day. This was probably the first time ever that any IIT or the incubator of any academic institution had installed a full-fledged manufacturing facility on campus.[1]

But then, these were far-from-normal times. The pandemic had changed it all. At the beginning of the pandemic, India was completely dependent on importing PPEs, masks, ventilators, HFNC machines, diagnostic kits, and so on. But because of worldwide demand, imports were neither easy[2] nor was the quality of such products dependable.[3] India had no option but to develop solutions on its own. At many science-and-technology teaching and research institutions across the country, even though only faculty members and a skeletal staff were available, the institutions rose to the occasion.

At IIT-K, the charge was led by the Director, Professor Abhay Karandikar, himself. He provided moral support to every project that was initiated by the IIT-K incubator, startups or faculty, and got actively involved in some of them. His sense of ownership and pride for the ventilator project became evident very early on in the journey. Even though the final outcome of the project was not predictable in late-March, he backed it unhesitatingly. He asked Amitabha to record a video on 25 March and showcased the nascent work on his social media handles. This provided the initial visibility the project needed among the large IIT-K alumni base, including Government of India's Principal Scientific Advisor, Professor K. VijayRaghavan who tweeted about it, which was then picked up by BBC.

Abhay Karandikar continued to remain our go-to person on several occasions when we hit a roadblock where his official intervention helped sort out matters. When the MOU negotiations with BDL were getting prolonged, he intervened by speaking directly with the chairman and MD of BDL. When our consignment of components was stuck in Singapore, he reached out to various government departments to try and find a solution.

Abhay Karandikar represents a generation of science and technology institution leaders who have a deep belief that the Indian market needs home-grown technologies and products relevant to our needs. Way back in 2012, he was lamenting the fact that India's telecom boom was largely on the back of imported equipment (as high as ₹54,765 crore in 2009–10 alone), mainly because foreign companies owned most of the IP in telecom.[4] In response to this, he championed the setting up of Telecommunications Standards Development

Society, India, (TSDSI) an autonomous standards development organization for telecom products in India. With this in place, Abhay and his colleagues from various IITs led the effort for including India-specific IP in the global standards for 5G. After considerable arm wrestling[5], TSDSI succeeded[6] in incorporating 'LMLC (Large Cell Low Mobility)' as part of International Telecommunications Union (ITU) 5G standard (officially called 5G 2020). Karandikar's team has also been working on 'Frugal 5G Networks' as part of IEEE (Institute of Electrical and Electronics Engineers, the world's largest technical professional organization) standard. Both these initiatives will help the expansion of broadband technology in rural India.[7]

Dr Ashwini Kumar Nangia, until recently the director of the National Chemical Laboratory (CSIR-NCL) in Pune, was another institution head working at the forefront. He spearheaded an interesting collaboration between his scientists and an enterprising firm, Chembond Polymers and Materials Ltd (CPML), to rapidly develop the naso-pharyngeal (NP) swabs used in Covid-19 testing. Until March, all NP swabs had been imported. NCL scientists procured some imported swabs, analyzed them, and worked out the underlying specifications quickly. 'We could do this analysis for Chembond in under three weeks – what would have otherwise taken them three months. We could deploy 100 man-years of scientific experience within a compressed time frame, and they got a six-month head start because of this,' says Dr Nangia.[8] Equipped with such medically acceptable specifications, Chembond quickly moved and executed the project. They did a mix-and-match with their suppliers and came up with about twenty permutations and combinations, of which they picked the most feasible ones to manufacture. The firm out-paced bigger players like Reliance and Johnson & Johnson, which failed to bring NP swabs to the market fast enough, even though they had made widely publicized announcements.[9] Using a cricket analogy to describe this outcome, Dr Nangia says, 'You cannot use a five-day test match strategy for a T20 game when time was of [the] essence. Even NCL scientists used a T20 attitude to get this done quickly.'

These examples are only a tiny fraction of the efforts undertaken by India's science-and-technology institutions during this period. But these initiatives were surprising given how much criticism the science-and-technology ecosystem had received for several decades.

Looking back at our history since independence, Indian science and technology institutions have rarely delivered on significant national priorities. One of these exceptional instances was very early after independence. The first general election in independent India was slated to be held in 1951–52. For a newly independent country the size of India, the caretaker government had a huge responsibility to ensure that Indians developed faith in democratic processes and national institutions. Holding a free and fair election was at the core of it all, and Sukumar Sen, the first chief election commissioner, was entrusted with the challenging aforementioned responsibility. He swung into action immediately and made a list of items that must be provided by the central government for the election: ballot boxes, paper seals for ballot boxes and indelible ink.[10]

In the absence of government-issued documents that could identify voters, indelible ink was necessary to prevent duplicate voting. The ink, once applied on the finger, penetrates the skin cells and produces a dark violet colour which remains indelible for up to ninety-six hours. Every voter was required to present their left forefinger to the presiding officer, demonstrate that there was no ink mark before they were given a ballot paper to cast their vote.

This was not a novel system; it had been used in many other countries, but India did not produce any indelible ink in 1947. And rather than import it from the British, which would have undermined the self-esteem of a newly independent nation,

India decided to make its own indelible ink for the first general election. The National Physical Laboratory (NPL) in Delhi was entrusted with this responsibility. NPL had a full-fledged ink development unit that had been producing a variety of inks including printing ink, and its team worked day and night to develop India's first indelible ink. The task of mass production was assigned to Mysore Paints and Varnish, a company owned by the then king of Mysore, Maharaja Nalvadi Krishnaraja Wodeyar. One of independent India's nascent science and technology institutions rose to the occasion and played its part in creating history towards a peaceful, free and fair election. Very few ex-British colonies could earn this distinction.

Barring a few notable achievements such as India's first indelible ink, the PARAM supercomputer, the space odyssey of Indian Space Research Organization, Indian science and technology institutions have been perceived as ivory towers, where scientists satisfy personal whims and fancies in the name of blue-sky scientific research at the expense of taxpayer money. In 2017–18, the cream of the Indian academic research-and-development ecosystem, including all the IITs and the research laboratories of different ministries, collectively filed a meagre 1,382 patents.[11] In comparison, 2,691 patents were filed in India by foreign applicants. In 2018, India topped the list of most abandoned patent applications (66.2%), indicating that not enough thought was given to actual market needs when undertaking work on these innovations.

There are two other reasons for these ailments. The first is that the readiness of such technologies is often too nascent to elicit any interest from industry partners. Secondly, a lack of communication between different stakeholders – technologists, public and private funding bodies, industrialists and the government – has hindered such development.

The big question now is: what changed during the pandemic?

Professor Ashutosh Sharma of IIT Kanpur is presently on lien to the government and serves as secretary of DST. According to him, 'There is no lack of talent or skill sets or infrastructure in India. What was needed was a direction which the pandemic provided, and that did the trick. The entire ecosystem – from R&D institutions to startups and the marketplace – worked with a shared and clear purpose.'[12] The same sentiment was echoed by Dr Renu Swarup, Secretary of Department of Biotechnology (DBT), who elaborated on how DBT catalyzed while the ecosystem players created a virtual network of dozens of industries, small and large, that acted together to ensure that the supply chain for diagnostic kits was entirely indigenized in a month's time.[13]

The other gap that was bridged during this period was the missing connect between the Indian science-and-technology ecosystem and the industry.[14] Previously, innovations from academic institutions were rarely picked up by any industry for further development and commercialization.[15] Also, during normal times, scientists and engineers often develop products that are of no immediate use. However, during the pandemic, the front page of every newspaper was screaming out 'needs' statements. It was clear that India needed a large supply of medical devices and equipment. As Professor Sharma has pointed out, this gave the academic ecosystem clear direction.

All science and technology funding bodies sprang to action almost immediately and simultaneously to ensure that the most promising efforts got funded promptly. The National Science and Technology Entrepreneurship Development Board (NSTEDB) is an organ under the DST, set up to promote knowledge-driven and technology-intensive enterprises. Under the leadership of Dr Anita Gupta, the CAWACH initiative was created almost overnight. It was anchored at IIT Bombay's technology business incubator (TBI) and had six satellite centres – all TBIs of various R&D institutions. On 6 April, it called for Covid-19 solutions that could be deployed within a few weeks. By 20 April, when the call was closed, 826 applications had been received.

The CAWACH centres had drafted a set of rules for conducting initial screenings. The applications were divided into subdisciplines (such as sterilizers and disinfectants; PPE and related products; medical equipment; diagnostics; contact tracing; and drugs and vaccines) and assigned to a group of CAWACH centres based on expertise. Each proposal was reviewed by three subject experts. The TBI teams and expert reviewers worked long hours to finish the first round of screening by 23 April. By 5 May, following an in-person interview-cum-demonstration in front of a panel of experts, fifty-one projects were awarded CAWACH grants. The funds were disbursed soon thereafter. The entire process was completed within a month, a record that will remain a matter of pride for years to come.

Similarly, the NSTEDB counterpart of the DBT is the Biotechnology Research Assistance Council (BIRAC). Efforts from BIRAC were being fronted by Dr Manish Diwan, head of Strategy Partnership and Entrepreneurship Development at BIRAC. It swung into action as early as mid-March.[17] A committee was set up to receive proposals, which were evaluated daily by a task force of experts. The initial focus was on products ready to be deployed within zero to three months of getting funded, in the domains of patient monitoring, rapid and cheap diagnosis of co-morbid conditions, and ICU equipment. By mid-April, BIRAC issued another call to solicit short-, mid- and long-term solutions for managing the pandemic. Within a month, nearly a 1,000 proposals were screened and seventy-one supported, including projects for vaccine research, novel diagnostics, cell-based therapies and re-purposing of drugs.

In all likelihood, when the pandemic broke, none of these Covid-19-related projects had budgetary provisions. For anyone familiar with the workings of Indian funding agencies, it is easy to imagine that heroic efforts must have been required to create such provisions so quickly.

Several autonomous R&D institutions under the government set up Covid diagnostic centres to ramp up tests, and India increased its total Covid testing from 0.76 tests per 1,000 of population in the first week of May, to around 44 tests per 1,000 of population by the first week of September. [18] At the time of writing this chapter in late September, India is testing more than a million per day, an enviable feat from the perspective of many countries. The achievement assumes significance when one takes into account that the UK has accumulated a massive testing backlog due to inadequate infrastructure.[19]

A scientist at the Indian Institute of Science (IISc), one of India's oldest and premier R&D institutes, developed a mobile testing unit that could conduct tests in remote areas with limited access to test laboratories. With the increase in testing data, it became possible to model the disease's progression accurately and use the data to plan strategic interventions. A collaborative effort between the Jawaharlal Nehru Centre for Advanced Scientific Research (JNCASR), IISc and IIT Bombay was backed by the DST to develop a national model for how Covid-19 would evolve in India, and the subsequent medical needs arising out of such projections.[20]

In mid-March, Principal Scientific Advisor to the Government of India, Dr K. VijayRaghavan, constituted the Task Force on Repurposing Drugs (TFORD) to speed up the lab-to-market journey. One of the two coordinators of TFORD, Dr V. Premnath, who is the head of NCL Innovations at CSIR-NCL and director at Venture Center, describes how they put together an advisory group of more than twenty-five experts to support the task force. 'We got the best experts into the team, including from the private sector – from medicinal chemistry, biology, those who did clinical trials, clinicians and doctors, people from the pharma industry, IP experts, and more. Everyone was generous with their time.'[21]

But can this new avatar be carried forward into peacetime?

A big word of reassurance about the future comes from Dr Renu Swarup. 'DBT will ensure that the collaborations that happened almost spontaneously during the pandemic are sustained so that the Indian academic R&D emerges as a fulcrum for the country's journey towards *atmanirbharta* or self-sustenance.'

Introducing a dose of realism, Dr Ashwini Nangia believes that not everything we learnt during the pandemic will be relevant. An active sportsperson in his younger days, he once again draws on a sports analogy. 'You can't use a sprint strategy for the long marathon.' Success will require work in two core areas. One, the government procedures that could be put on the back burner during Covid times cannot be so in normal times. Two, getting people to work together for a short period was possible even if they had philosophical differences, but that's harder in the longer term and requires a change in mindsets.

But mindsets are indeed changing across the board, and that should make us hopeful. Especially since the government, the biggest backer of incubators, is itself becoming very proactive and supportive of innovative ventures.

KEY TAKEAWAYS

India's science and technology institutions rose to the occasion during the Covid-19 pandemic.

- Historically, scientists and researchers at India's premier institutions have focused their energies on problems far removed from the nation's pressing needs.
- During the pandemic, many of them reoriented quickly to help develop solutions that would help fight the pandemic.
- There are reasons to believe that the change in mindset and collaborative approach seen during the pandemic can be sustained in future.

STARTER KIT (FOR SCIENCE AND TECHNOLOGY INSTITUTIONS, GOVERNMENT AGENCIES AND PRIVATE SECTOR)

STEP 1: Government and private sector should periodically publish clear 'problem statements', focused on significant issues that require innovative solutions from inventors and researchers at our science and technology Institutions. iDEX (Innovations for Defence Excellence) is a good example of how the Defence Ministry has invited co-creation of innovation and technology development in the defence and aerospace sectors.

STEP 2: Funding, in significant measure, through grants, debt, or equity should be aligned to work in these areas.

STEP 3: Successes should frequently be publicly showcased and celebrated. This will further create an upward spiral of interest and participation.

Notes

1. Malhotra, Abhinav. 'IIT-Kanpur starts production of N95 and N99 Masks to fight Covid.' *Times of India*, 19 June 2020. https://timesofindia.indiatimes.com/city/kanpur/iit-kanpur-starts-production-of-n95-and-n99-masks-to-fight-covid/articleshow/76453991.cms.
2. Thacker, Teena and Anandita Singh Mankotia. 'Tens of Thousands of Chinese PPE Kits Fail India Safety Test.' *Economic Times*, 16 April 2020. https://economictimes.indiatimes.com/industry/healthcare/biotech/tens-of-thousands-of-chinese-ppe-kits-fail-india-safety-test/articleshow/75171817.cms?from=mdr.
3. 'India Coronavirus: Rapid Testing Paused over China Kit Issues.' *BBC*, 22 April 2020. https://www.bbc.com/news/world-asia-india-52378265.
4. Karandikar, Abhay. 'India Needs Umbrella Body on Telecom Standards to Foster Creation of IPR and Develop Indigenous Products.' *Economic Times*, [Updated on] 16 August 2012. https://economictimes.indiatimes.com/opinion/et-commentary/india-needs-

umbrella-body-on-telecom-standards-to-foster-creation-of-ipr-and-develop-indigenous-products/articleshow/15510374.cms.

5. 'India Makes its Maiden Entry into 5G Standards, Pisses off Big Telecoms.' *Communications Today*, 14 February 2019. https://www.communicationstoday.co.in/india-makes-its-maiden-entry-into-5g-standards-pisses-off-big-telecoms/.
6. ITU. 'ITU Completes Evaluation for Global Affirmation of IMT-2020 Technologies.' Press release, 26 November 2020. https://www.itu.int/en/mediacentre/Pages/pr26-2020-evaluation-global-affirmation-imt-2020-5g.aspx?fbclid=IwAR3onAP7G5-DKsQxjzv4lrc2HSw5_mbV9xgSkBQ5gpmz2QVeTIrJFEAvPJA.
7. *World Intellectual Property Indicators 2019*. Geneva: WIPO, 2019 https://www.wipo.int/edocs/pubdocs/en/wipo_pub_941_2019.pdf.
8. Dr Ashwini Nangia's interview with the authors.
9. 'Made-in-India Coronavirus Test Swabs to Cost Only One-tenth of Imported Ones.' *Hindu*, 17 May 2020. https://www.thehindu.com/news/national/india-brings-down-corona-test-swab-price-to-one-tenth/article31607194.ece.
10. Election Commision of India. 'Report on the First General Elections in India 1951–52. Volume I (General).' 1955. p. 95.
11. WIPO. *World Intellectual Property Indicators 2019*. Geneva: World Intellectual Property Organization. https://www.wipo.int/edocs/pubdocs/en/wipo_pub_941_2019.pdf.
12. Dr Ashutosh Sharma's interview with the authors.
13. Dr Renu Swarup's interview with the authors.
14. 'Transforming Science and Technology in India,' in *Economic Survey 2017–18 Volume 1*. January 2018. pp. 119–130. http://mofapp.nic.in:8080/economicsurvey/pdf/119-130_Chapter_08_ENGLISH_Vol_01_2017-18.pdf.
15. 'Commercialization of Indigenously Developed Technologies.' CSIR-Indian Institute of Petroleum. https://www.inae.in/storage/2018/12/August-2015-Commercialization-of-Indigenously-Developed-Technologies-by-M.O.-GARG.pdf. https://www.inae.in/storage/2018/12/August-2015-Commercialization-of-Indigenously-Developed-Technologies-by-M.O.-GARG.pdf.
16. Dr Anita Gupta's interview with the authors.
17. Dr Manish Diwan's interview with the authors.

18. 'Total Covid-19 Tests per 1,000 People.' Our World in Data. https://ourworldindata.org/grapher/full-list-cumulative-total-tests-per-thousand?time=2020-02-20..latestHe9e9.
19. 'UK Faces Backlog of Nearly 200,000 Covid-19 Tests in Government Labs.' *Financial Times*, 13 September 2020. https://www.ft.com/content/45a559bd-ec00-426b-9f05-ac962ba49375.
20. Nair, Lakshmipriya. 'Mathematical Modelling Can Enable the Entire Gamut of Decision-makers to Make Informed Choices.' *Express Healthcare*, 23 April 2020. https://www.expresshealthcare.in/covid19-updates/mathematical-modelling-can-enable-the-entire-gamut-of-decision-makers-to-make-informed-choices/419219/.
21. Dr V. Premnath's interview with the authors.

23

The Government Gets It, Mostly

On 25 June 2020, Amitabha was sorting through his inbox when he spotted a strange email in which he had been copied. It was from the High Commission of India in Singapore, thanking Rahul Patel of the IIT-K task force for making a payment quickly, with a request for an additional payment of twenty Singapore dollars.

The email was the culmination of a fascinating drama that had played out in early April, when various arms of the government had come together as divine help to support the task force that was praying for a miracle to happen. This was on 1 April, and we had just then heard that DHL – the big global player in logistics – which had promised to fly in our consignment of components from Singapore to India, had backed out at the last moment because of the lockdown in India. It was no April Fool's Day joke either. We were now really clutching at every straw to bring in this consignment of components from the Singapore-based supplier before Singapore went into lockdown on 3 April. Every other logistics provider we contacted said it would take more than two weeks to deliver the items, and that too wasn't certain. For us to stay on course to develop the V110, the first version of our ventilator, we desperately needed to get the shipment out. We began knocking at every door – the

Cabinet Secretariat, the Department for Promotion of Industry and Internal Trade (DPIIT), even the Ministry of Electronics and Information Technology.

It was at this time that Invest India, India's national investment promotion and facilitation agency, appeared as a saviour and took over the entire coordination for the shipment. Chandrima Sinha, VP of Invest India, coordinated with Rahul Patel in the task force as they contacted the Ministry of External Affairs and the Ministry of Civil Aviation to see if an Air India flight could bring in the consignment. A flight was confirmed for 4 April, but this route fell through at the last minute as our consignment was not big enough. Invest India then reached out to the Singapore Embassy in Delhi to check if Singapore Airlines had planned any special flights. As luck would have it, there was indeed one flight coming from Singapore to India to take stranded citizens back home. Invest India requested Singapore Airlines that our consignment be put on that flight. To deliver the consignment to the aircraft, we were directed to a Singapore freight forwarder – Speedmark – on 8 April. Speedmark needed to be paid in advance, but because banks were not operating at full capacity during the lockdown, it was impossible to remit money overseas from India quickly. Invest India stepped in once again and reached out to the High Commission of India in Singapore, which agreed to provide a payment guarantee to Speedmark on our behalf. When Singapore Airlines flight SQ 406 flew out on 9 April with our consignment and landed in Mumbai that night, we breathed a sigh of relief.

The payment to Speedmark, for which the Indian High Commission had so generously stood as a guarantor, was immediately remitted thereafter. The email Amitabha had received on 25 June was to point out that Speedmark had asked for an additional twenty-Singapore-dollar payment to cover the service charges the bank had deducted for the wire transfer. We were able to transfer the sum within a day.

The whole saga played out like a nail-biter. All the government agencies helped us without really knowing who we were. All they knew was that a group of Indians were making desperate efforts to save some lives, and the agencies rose to the occasion to essay a chapter in their history that had never been written before.

Both the centre and the state governments did many things well during the crisis. To a large extent, this was possible because of the foundation that had been laid out in the past five to six years. The launch of Make in India (2014) and Startup India (2016), and the revival of a defunct Invest India (2014) helped sensitize the bureaucracy and make them business friendly. There were indeed some areas where the government fell short. Part of this could be attributed to an evolutionary learning process for bureaucrats, and part of it is equally indicative of the structural gaps in the government's working that may be harder to fix.

The government's structure does not make it easy for it to work with energetic startups, but several individuals within the government do so instinctively and willingly. At the top of this list is V. Venugopal Reddy, Principal Secretary of Industries and Mining in Maharashtra. The Nocca founders were introduced to him by the president of the Mumbai chapter of IIT Kanpur's alumni association. Reddy became our go-to person every time the team was stuck while needing to move software engineers from Nanded or Mumbai to Pune, or for permissions to transport crucial components by road. In Pune, Rubal Agarwal, Additional Municipal Commissioner, stepped in on several occasions. The ventilator project could not have been pulled off but for the timely help from many such people in government across the country.

Task force member Padmaja Ruparel, also the president of IAN, was often at the forefront of seeking such help. She found that a lot of these efforts worked because someone knew someone in the government. 'It's completely person-dependent, and hasn't been structurally fixed as an enabling framework,' she says. She thought it would have been easier if the PM's call had been followed up by the appointment of a nodal agency or person at the PMO, DPIIT, or the Finance Ministry. Someone who could have acted as a single window to get roadblocks cleared for Covid-related products and services.

Fortunately, some government agencies that had cut their teeth over the past decade sprang into action quickly and were able to mobilize various parts of the ecosystem they had influence over. Dr Ashutosh Sharma, Secretary of the DST, is happy about how his ministry could activate multiple organizations simultaneously, all in pursuit of the same objective. The Science and Engineering Research Board, one of the agencies he oversees, issued calls for scientific proposals aimed at long-term solutions, while the entire incubator ecosystem was triggered by NSTEDB to provide immediate solutions. 'Even NGOs were roped in,' he says.[1]

MyLabs, the startup that developed the first approved RT-PCR diagnostic kit from India, got substantial financial support from Technology Development Board (TDB), yet another agency overseen by Dr Sharma's DST. Under normal circumstances, such a large investment would have taken much longer due to due diligence needs. Here, the process was not short-circuited, but all relevant sections of TDB and DST worked round the clock to ensure the timely release of funds.

BIRAC is one of the most nimble-footed government agencies. Set up as a Section-8 public sector enterprise by the Department of Biotechnology in 2012 to catalyze the creation of a $100 billion bioeconomy in India, BIRAC had already earned its spurs in recent years through its work with startups and SMEs. As early as 19 March, BIRAC announced the creation of a Covid-19 research consortium and invited companies to apply if they had solutions for diagnostics, vaccines, novel therapeutics, and so on. It backed it up with another announcement promising fast-tracked review and funding support. Under the fast-track mechanism, if someone had a solution ready that just needed funding, they could get up to ₹5 crore within two days.

Not surprisingly, a big part of BIRAC's focus during the pandemic was diagnostic kits. 'The virus was new and there was no tool available to detect it. We needed diagnostic kits fast. Until then, they were only imported. We were paying hefty amounts to get tests done. The research and startup community took it as a challenge,' says Dr Manish Diwan, head of Strategy Partnership and Entrepreneurship Development at BIRAC.[2] Five startups and SMEs came forth, but most of them depended on nearly 70% imports, while the initial cost of kits was ₹1,200. BIRAC pushed them to indigenize. The latest RT-PCR kits now cost between ₹120 and ₹150 and are 100% indigenized.

BIRAC received 1,200 applications for various solutions. All of them were screened, reviewed, approved and disbursed online in record time thanks to its staff burning the midnight oil. In all, seventy-five Covid products were funded (including the research for a vaccine) for a sum ranging from ₹15 lakh to ₹50 crore. Within three to four months, several ideas translated themselves to products on the shelf, and India made itself self-reliant with respect to many products, PPEs and masks being two prime examples.

While DST and BIRAC were quickly nurturing promising solutions, Invest India, as the secretariat for the government's empowered group for essential medical supplies, was rapidly identifying suppliers and stocks for products ranging from ventilators to PPE kits and masks. It worked with logistics providers whenever there were bottlenecks, as it did with us when it stepped in to help us bring our consignment from Singapore.

Clearly, several government agencies put in superhuman efforts and displayed a 'can do' attitude during the pandemic.

This enabled startups and bigger companies to achieve seemingly impossible results. Can this approach be carried forward into the new normal? What will it take to make that happen?

We asked three people who intensively engage with the government for their insights.

Padmaja Ruparel has in recent years seen specific initiatives come to life, for example, the resolution of the angel tax issue, startup certification, ranking of states, and fund of funds (a mega fund that invests in other funds instead of investing directly in companies; under the Startup India programme, the government created a fund of funds for startups). All these initiatives saw the light of day only because some proactive senior bureaucrat had championed them.

Similarly, as CEO of the IIMCIP, Dr Subhrangshu Sanyal has worked closely with state governments in West Bengal, Assam, Meghalaya, Mizoram and Arunachal Pradesh. His experience is similar to Padmaja's. 'When senior leaders and bureaucrats take the lead, it makes a big difference. The Nest, Assam's fantastic incubator in Guwahati, came up because the Industries Secretary of the time believed in it, and his successor backed it as well,' says Dr Sanyal.[3] It is no different in other states. Often there's a gap between a visionary senior bureaucrat (such bureaucrats are from the Indian Administrative Services) and junior officers (who are often from the state cadre). But IIMCIP's success could be achieved because they have worked with all levels of the bureaucracy. Junior levels is where implementation takes place. IAS officers move on to other roles, but the state cadre is permanent.

Dr Nikhil Agarwal, CEO of IIT Kanpur's incubator, has worked for the governments of Andhra Pradesh and Maharashtra in the recent past. In addition, as a senior advisor with FIICI BISNET, he has also provided guidance to the West Bengal, Uttar Pradesh and Uttarakhand governments. He has vivid memories of how well things were going in Andhra Pradesh while working with erstwhile chief minister Chandrababu Naidu and his chief secretary. Among other things, Nikhil had sought and received approval for setting up a cyber security park in Tirupati. But when a new chief secretary came in, everything fell flat. 'While the government is a collective institution, it is really a collection of individuals underneath. To make headway, you need to find and work with the right individual[s]. Second, if you demonstrate passion and intent, and the government develops trust over time, they'll back you.' Nikhil's closing words have a biting reality. 'The government is worse than a bank. Because they manage people's money and receive thousands of proposals, they have to say "no" to most. They say "yes" when you show conviction and develop trust.'[4]

The good news is that many government agencies that were active when the Covid-19 pandemic hit India are building on the momentum. Dr Ashutosh Sharma is confident that the new science-and-technology policy will bring industry and academia closer with provisions for joint funding where industry–academia collaboration projects of national importance may be funded up to 90% by the government. He is also happy about the fact that the governing body for the National Mission on Interdisciplinary Cyber Physical Systems (NM-ICPS) will now be chaired by an industry leader, Kris Gopalakrishnan, rather than by a scientist or an academician.

Dr Manish Diwan believes that BIRAC can carry forward all the recent learnings, especially the ability to access experts quickly through online meetings so that local innovations can be empowered strongly. 'We're importing 85% of our medical equipment. That needs to be reduced and replaced with domestic products. We need to customize solutions for Indian context by getting rid of frills and fancies. Our devices need to work under conditions of poor electricity and internet. Similar solutions can be taken to eighty countries that are non-regulated markets,' Dr Diwan spells out.

A big step in this direction was taken in India's 2020 Budget. The actual budgetary clauses, as below, are in typical government lingo:

'63 (2). Knowledge Translation Clusters would be set up across different technology sectors including new and emerging areas.

63 (3). For designing, fabrication and validation of proof of concept, and further scaling up Technology Clusters, harbouring such test beds and small-scale manufacturing facilities would be established.'[5]

In plain English, the government announced the creation of ten technology propellers, to take ideas from concept to pilot, and five manufacturing zones by 2025. We should expect to see at least two technology propellors and one manufacturing zone come up each year from hereon.

Indian startups and companies should be happy on this score. Padmaja Ruparel's wish list, as a spokesperson for the startup ecosystem, is on similar lines. She would like to see a greater risk appetite within various government committees that decide on investing in startups. While industry experts have been brought into the committees in recent years, what is still missing is an enabling structure that helps investment committees take some seemingly risky but robust bets on promising startups without having to worry about vigilance inquiries later on.

Vijaya Kumar Ivaturi, the author of *The Manual for Indian Startups*, has one big ask and a few smaller ones. The big ask is what he calls a 'demand-side enablement',[5] that is, revamping the government procurement model to make it easier for startups to get business from various government projects. He recommends all large infrastructure projects that have a consortium-led model to bid, win and deliver should mandatorily include one startup or more in the consortium to bring in both innovation and completeness to the solution. The startup in such cases would not merely be a subcontractor to the principal bidder, but actually own a part of the contract. A financial institution like SIDBI would need to provide some support to the startup so that it can remain in good health until project revenues start flowing in.

His other asks, though smaller in scope of effort, can make a huge difference. The first is about the diversity and complexity of various government schemes that make it hard for startups to decipher them. Our incubators, as key interfaces, need to develop both an information system and a tool that can help startups understand the full range of schemes across central and state governments, and provide help in writing these proposals. The second, again a fair ask, is about how the eligibility criteria keeps changing across central and state governments with respect to the definition of startups and MSMEs. There is also a variance by sector.

All in all, notwithstanding some disappointments, the recent approach of the government holds out reasons for optimism. If this new normal triumphs over the traditional Indian normal, there is no force that can stop us from taking big strides towards making Atmanirbhar Bharat a reality and meeting the rising expectations of a new generation of youth across the country.

KEY TAKEAWAYS

Some big strides have been taken by the government, but a few more are required.

- During the pandemic, several government agencies and officers were proactive in supporting startups and companies creating Covid-related products and services.
- With these successes under their belt, the government agencies appear determined to sustain the momentum in the post-Covid age as well.
- Incubators would greatly benefit by learning how to work with different levels of the bureaucracy within both the central and state governments.

- Two ways in which the government can plug gaps are by creating an enabling framework that encourages risks, while investing in startups and revamping the procurement model to allow startups to get business from the government.

STARTER KIT

STEP 1: The government has a range of funding schemes (grant, debt, equity) for startups and many of these originate from the National Science and Technology Development Board (NSTEDB), an agency created by the DST, or from BIRAC, an agency created by the DBT. These schemes cover the requirements of technology startups all the way from ideation to prototype development to commercialization. These schemes are often hard to understand or keep track of. The best way to access this valuable pool is through one of the more than 150 technology business incubators or 50 bioincubators across the country.

STEP 2: The government is an active regulator in many categories. In sectors like healthcare or fintech, it is best to have board members or advisors or employees who can understand and help the startups navigate through the regulatory maze. Not doing so can lead to both delays and higher costs.

STEP 3: The government is also a big buyer of products and services. Tapping into this revenue opportunity requires a two-fold strategy. First, get familiar with the Government eMarketplace (GeM), which now has a specific 'GeM Startup Runway', to participate in e-procurement. Secondly, hire team member(s) who are experienced in selling to the government sector.

Notes

1. Dr Ashutosh Sharma's interview with the authors.
2. Dr Manish Diwan's interview with the authors.
3. Dr Subhrangshu Sanyal's interview with the authors.
4. Dr Nikhil Agarwal's interview with the authors.

5. 'Budget 2020: Full Text of Nirmala Sitharaman's Budget Speech.' *Mint*, 1 February 2020. https://www.livemint.com/budget/news/budget-2020-full-text-of-nirmala-sitharaman-s-budget-speech-11580547114996.html.
6. Vijaya Kumar Ivaturi's interview with the authors.

24

Small-town Talent

Twenty-four-year-old Tushar Agarwal had a quiet swagger even during his high-school days in Mathura, Uttar Pradesh. He loved coding, and during one of his practical exams, he wrote some correct code, but in a way that his teacher did not understand. This Computer Science teacher, who had joined the school only recently, insisted on not giving him full marks. The matter got escalated and reached the principal, and another Computer Science teacher was asked to arbitrate by reviewing the answer sheet. Tushar was awarded full marks and the original teacher was admonished. This was the small-town confidence we saw in full bloom when he engaged in those vigorous technical debates with the two guru–mentors in the task force – Padma Bhushan Ajai Chowdhry and Padma Shri Saurabh Srivastava.

Now based in Pune, Tushar and his buddies – the founders of Nocca, who come from Shahdol (Madhya Pradesh) and Kanpur (Uttar Pradesh) respectively – represent just the tip of the iceberg. Their success with the ventilator project is part of the big startup wave that is sweeping across non-metro India. Coincidentally, most members of the task force – including many senior mentors – have grown up in small towns.

The startup phenomenon has moved beyond the traditional centres of Bengaluru, Delhi-NCR, Mumbai, Chennai and Hyderabad to smaller towns. What television did for cricket, the spread of 4G – including access to YouTube – did for Indian startups. At a startup event in Patna in October 2018, Srikant was accosted by five students who had been enthusiastic enough to undertake a two-night train journey from Bhilwara in Rajasthan to Patna for the event.

The pandemic, especially the remote working and collaborative tools that have come into play because of it, has accelerated this phenomenon. Location became a non-issue during the lockdown. Technology allowed the Nocca founders in Pune to talk to mentors in Delhi, Dehradun, Bengaluru, New York and California. In normal circumstances, the two founders would have at best had quarterly face-to-face meetings and monthly calls with a few of the mentors. There wouldn't be anything as intense as a daily ninety-minute call for three months at a stretch.

Viren Rasquinha, the CEO of Olympic Gold Quest (OGQ), a not-for-profit organization that identifies and nurtures promising athletes, sees the same phenomenon in sports.[1] India's big badminton hope for the future comes from Lakshya Sen, ranked twenty-seventh in the World Badminton Federation's (BWF) men's singles rankings.[2] If Covid-19 hadn't come in the way, he could have taken a shot at getting into the top fifteen.[3]

Lakshya is just nineteen. He's from Almora in Uttarakhand, and his nascent talent was spotted by Bengaluru's Prakash Padukone Academy when he was just ten years old.[4] OGQ immediately stepped in to support his training and preparation. OGQ supports 210 players across badminton, boxing, shooting, archery and wrestling – individual sports – where India has talent and has done well, are the country's medal hopes in future Olympics tournaments. It is remarkable that like Lakshya, 90% of the OGQ players are from non-metro cities. 'Most wrestlers are from Haryana, boxers are from Manipur and Haryana, and shooters from across India, as also the badminton players,' says Rasquinha.

Rasquinha thinks athletes from non-metros possess not just the talent, but also the fire and the desire to be the best, and continuously learn and improve their skills. He speculates that these youngsters have greater risk appetites because they have fewer educational and career opportunities in their towns, and sport is a risky venture to start with. Most interestingly, also a useful lesson for the startup world, Viren finds that girls are far more talented and resilient than boys.

A similar trend started in cricket two decades ago. Cricket commentator and journalist Harsha Bhogle says, 'With the onset of satellite TV showing national and international cricket, ambition was stoked in small towns, and knowledge spread rapidly too. Youngsters were suddenly seeing the likes of Warne, Ponting and Kallis in action and emulating their batting or bowling actions.'[5]

We should expect to see many more startups from small towns now, especially from towns where an IIT or NIT (there are twenty-three IITs and thirty-one NITs currently) can become a local hub for techies to congregate. Aspiring entrepreneurs from anywhere in India – be it Leh, Aizawl, Raipur, Udaipur or Thrissur – can engage with incubators, accelerators, mentors and investors like never before. Almost every member of the ventilator task force has already been roped in to remotely mentor other startups. Such location-agnostic initiatives which can support small-town startups are here to stay. As part of his incubator engagements, Srikant has mentored startups from Bardhaman (Aegipan), Guwahati (Zerund), Jaipur (Module Innovation), Yernagudem (Kritsnam), Nagaon (3D Selfie) and Pune (BioPrime).

Covid-19 and technology made everyone become comfortable with working in a location-agnostic manner. But some big companies had tried this out even before the pandemic. Tiger Tyagarajan took over as CEO of Genpact in 2011. Soon after, he announced that the company's top leaders must be closer to customers across nine cities in the world rather than being based in their Gurgaon headquarters. He also abolished the concept of a headquarter. The company embraced the proposal, its quantum of travel reduced, and customers loved it as well. Today, Covid-19 has reinforced the need to travel even less for a company like Genpact. Tiger expects a change with respect to customers and talent as well from hereon. Customers may no longer expect service providers to travel for minor meetings. The talent paradigm will also change and will not be constrained by location.[6]

Remote collaboration products like WebEx, MS Teams, Skype Business, Zoom, Slack, BlueJeans have been around for a while now. The pandemic has made them more mainstream by making them essential for everyone. Palo Alto investor Sunil Singh is optimistic that it will not just make it easy for companies to access new talent pools, but also make the customer sales process easier for startups based in India, even in the small towns. 'Remote sales teams will become more mainstream, and they will no longer have to compete with on-ground relationship-based sales teams who can wine and dine and build trust with the customer,' he argues.[7]

However, some of the challenges of non-metro towns will not go away. A lot of the engineering (or medical) talent from non-premier institutes, especially the private ones, will need to be retrained before they can create a startup, or join one. Without being technically strong, they will not be able to inspire confidence among investors and mentors. Dr Gautam Ahuja of Cornell University, who has seen smaller cities in the US struggle to compete with bigger metropolitan areas as hubs of economic activity, reminds us that other kinds of support are also important: business infrastructure, digital and physical connectivity, quality of life, attracting high-quality talent and simplified government regulations.[8]

Language is another important issue in India. While speaking at the Patna startup event, Srikant switched to Hindi after realizing many aspiring entrepreneurs in the audience hailed from smaller towns in Bihar and were not comfortable with English. The change in language made an immediate impact, and audience interactions improved dramatically. This learning was heightened even further during a startup event in Aizawl, Mizoram, where Srikant was part of a jury evaluating the finalists of a state-wide startup challenge. Several finalists created their slides in English but spoke in Mizo. Srikant and two other non-Mizo jury members relied on the English slides and on Mizo-to-English translations offered by the Mizo jury members, when required. Without these innovations, Srikant would have missed some very inventive ideas. Srikant also dubbed his Chalo Startup video series in the Mizo language for a presentation to the chief minister and other dignitaries at the plenary session.

Such challenges notwithstanding, we are clearly at the cusp of a take-off point for smaller cities in India. Over the past few years, we have seen promising startups – like Phool from Kanpur, which converts temple-waste to consumer products; Sattuz from Madhubani, Bihar, which makes desi superfoods; Aegipan from West Bengal, which is a micro-entrepreneur network that helps goat farmers with animal husbandry; and BioPrime from Pune that has created several disruptive innovations in agriculture – make impressive progress. Imagine what such entrepreneurs can do in a post-Covid world if location barriers are demolished. Watch out for many more startup success stories from non-metros in the post-pandemic world when the war clouds of Covid are gone.

KEY TAKEAWAYS

There is untapped startup potential in non-metro India.

- The startup wave has reached non-metro cities and towns and remote locations across India.
- Remote working tools and change of habit during the pandemic have made it possible for startups to connect with the mainstream, especially mentors, easily.
- Several measures will be required to harness and nurture this explosion of startup talent, including systematic talent identification, skill enhancement, infrastructure, mentoring and language sensitivities.

STARTER KIT (FOR GOVERNMENT AGENCIES AND INCUBATORS)

STEP 1: Create programmes that identify promising startup talent across the length and breadth of the state/country. Many states already do this, but these programmes often tend to skim the surface by focusing on aspirants from top-tier engineering colleges and bigger cities. Going down to every district and evangelizing this is extremely crucial. North-eastern states like Mizoram and Meghalaya have done good work in this sphere by laying out multi-year initiatives and executing them well.

STEP 2: Systematic talent identification will need to be backed by structured multi-functional mentoring, skill enhancements (especially in tech and marketing), access to larger markets and local language support. The most promising venture ideas with national or global potential will need access to investors, accelerators and incubators in the bigger metro cities.

STEP 3: A majority of entrepreneurs from these locations are likely to create products or services that either address local needs or can achieve only limited scale, and therefore may not be of interest to mainstream VCs or even bigger angel investor networks. But these entrepreneurs will certainly create local jobs and livelihoods. To meet their financing needs, state government grants and loans will have a big role to play (₹10–25 lakh per venture). In addition, each state will need at least one local angel investing network comprising philanthropists and businessmen. The government could provide matching amounts in such cases.

Notes

1. Viren Rasquinha's interview with the authors.
2. 'Lakshya Sen: Ranking History: Profile.' BWF Fansite. https://bwfbadminton.com/player/68870/lakshya-sen/ranking-history.
3. '"I Was on Course for Top-15": Lakshya Sen Counts Losses amid Covid-19 Lockdown.' *Indian Express*, 27 April 2020. https://indianexpress.com/article/sports/badminton/lakshya-sen-ranking-titles-losses-covid-19-lockdown-6381722/.
4. Ninan, Susan. 'Lakshya Marks His Arrival in the Big Boys' League.' *ESPIN*, 12 March 2020. https://www.espn.in/badminton/story/_/id/28891957/all-england-open-lakshya-sen-marks-arrival-big-boys-league-gladiatorial-battle-vs-viktor-axelsen.
5. Harsha Bhogle's interview with the authors.
6. Tiger Tyagrajan's interview with the authors.
7. Sunil Singh's interview with the authors.
8. Dr Gautam Ahuja's interview with the authors.

25

Wartime Success vs Peacetime Success

Is a big crisis a necessary condition for people, teams or nations to put their best foot forward and become united by a common and higher purpose? Is there a common success formula for winning a war, a bitterly fought match, or a battle against a pandemic? Can this formula then be replicated during 'peacetime'?

The best explanation comes from two healthcare veterans who were part of the task force that helped Nocca. Rakesh Bhargava and Sanjiv Verma had separately run large organizations for the better part of their lives. Rakesh, who was Chairman at Fresenius Kabi Oncology, a German healthcare company, pinpoints unambiguous and common goals without any personal agenda as the key reasons for the success of the ventilator project in getting a great product designed, certified, accepted by doctors, manufactured and made available in the market – all in record time. 'All of us in the task force worked with the goal of making a great product and pass the test at Nirman Bhavan (Ministry of Health and Family Welfare).'

Similarly, ex-Managing Director of Baxter India, an American multinational healthcare company, Sanjiv Verma provides a more evocative description. 'The bridegroom was Nocca Robotics and getting the groom safely to the *mandap* was everyone's objective!' Each member of the task force brought their expertise and experience, while respecting others for their fortes, and everyone rolled up their sleeves to do the work. It was important to have a team of doers rather than talkers.

A similar shared feeling was at play during the Manhattan Project, the code name for the mission to create a nuclear bomb in secret facilities across the US at the height of World War II. Theoretical physicist Richard Feynman was a doctoral student at Princeton University when he joined the project. Scientific Director Robert Oppenheimer was worried that a group of IBM engineers, who had been co-opted into the project for computing support, were making slow progress. He asked Feynman to figure out why. Feynman realized that the engineers had been put in barracks and told nothing. 'They were merely coming each day to work on IBM machines – punching holes, numbers that they didn't understand.'[1] He concluded that 'these technical guys need[ed] to know what we're doing'. The engineers had to be given the big picture!

Oppenheimer went and got special permission from security officers for Feynman to brief the engineers. As soon as Feynman did so, they all got excited. 'We're fighting a war! They knew what the numbers meant. They knew what they were working on.' This led to a total transformation in their attitude. 'They didn't need any supervising and started inventing ways of doing it better.' The crisis of a war and a sense of national duty had brought out the best in these engineers.

Former Indian hockey captain Viren Rasquinha has vivid memories of the 2001 Junior Men's Hockey World Cup that India eventually won.[2] India had been the runner-up at the previous World Cup, so it was a huge shock when the next time they lost a crucial group-stage match to Australia and were placed at the precipice of the tournament. To stay in contention, India had to beat the Dutch in their next must-win game, while the results of other games also had to be in their favour. Coach Rajinder Singh charged his team up by invoking national pride, saying that Indian hockey could never be revived if they couldn't win that crucial match.[3] The reinvigorated Indian team beat the Netherlands 4–3, going on to win two more games to become tournament champions. A temporary crisis and national pride had made all the difference!

The pandemic took India by surprise, as it did the rest of the world. But diverse stakeholders such as the government, civil society, corporations, universities and research institutions came together to fight the virus. A month into the lockdown, as the migrant worker crisis became known, Professor Madhushree Nanda Agarwal, who teaches at Management Development Institute, Gurgaon, and her spouse volunteered to work for the Gurgaon Nagrik Ekta Manch, a volunteer-led civil society organization that helped thousands of people in acute financial distress in Gurgaon. This virtual network of volunteers, with no bank accounts or registered offices and only a social media presence, quickly mobilized resources to deliver cooked food and dry rations to lakhs of workers.[4] Similarly, the liquor company Diageo India produced hand sanitizers in five days, a product they had never made before. For Managing Director Anand Kripalu and his team, it was a moment of pride that came with a higher purpose and a lower cost of failure.[5]

Some of India's biggest transformational moments have come during moments of crisis – the Green Revolution, the White Revolution, even liberalization. People tend to wholeheartedly back change during such moments. Behavioural scientist Dr Leena Chatterjee of IIM-C finds that a crisis puts us into a 'fight' mode whereby we generate more energy and creativity in tackling a common enemy. A clear focus helps drive the activity. Also, when we feel overwhelmed or helpless, we are more willing to collaborate with others.[6] Similarly, in his book *Accidental India*, journalist–analyst Shankkar Aiyar argues that the major turning points in India's history were not the result of foresight or careful planning, but rather accidental consequences of major crises that had to be resolved at any cost. Aiyar uses the principles of physics to explain this: 'Newton's law prevails across sectors – society, politics and business. When status quo becomes a comfort zone, it requires an external force to force action. What makes people come together is the spectre of risk. The threat factor takes away the luxury of procrastination – the hope that the crisis will go away with time. Coalition of interests enables collaboration.'[7]

Is it therefore possible to create similar personal and collective enthusiasm during normal times as long as there is a higher purpose, clear goals and a leadership-plus-organizational structure, however informal or formal? This question intrigued the task force members. Could the ventilator experience be replicated at other promising startups? And could this model become an integral part of 'peacetime' engagement with startups? How can a similar sense of purpose and spirit of collaboration be achieved during normal times? Could Indians come together and solve some of our significant socio-economic challenges? And could Indian companies leverage their skills and frugal business models to scale themselves globally?

Tiger Tyagarajan has two prescriptions for uniting people behind a higher purpose during normal times.[8] His first recommendation is to create a crisis within the enterprise, 'a burning platform' as he describes it. This is an approach mastered by Jack Welch at GE, a company where Tiger worked for over ten years. Corporate folklore has it that every time Welch felt his team at GE was getting complacent, he would invoke a real or imaginary crisis, for example, 'Japanese and Korean companies are out to eat into our business. We need to do something fast.' Tiger's second recommendation is to create and set a goal that's outlandish because during normal times we tend to impose artificial constraints on ourselves that limit our audacity. At Genpact, which provides finance and accounting as one of its services, Tiger says, 'When a client asks if we can close their books of accounts within three weeks instead of four, we ask ourselves why can't we do it in forty-eight hours?'

We put together advice from the experts about creating successful outcomes during non-crisis periods to combine it into a simple five-point formula:

1) Urgency: a clear deadline or time period within which a specific problem needs to be solved plays an important role in getting team members to think fast and smart.
2) Idea: whether simple or hugely disruptive, ideas bring people together. An idea that the team develops for solving the problem creates a sense of purpose.
3) Champion(s): an individual or group of individuals who lead from the front, get their hands dirty and provide direction when required.
4) Safe environment: where people can participate as equals and collaborate safely with a spirit of openness, unlike a dog-eat-dog work environment.
5) Motivation and momentum: regular calendarized interactions ensure that the train stays on the rails and keeps moving, enabling each team member to contribute actively and seek help when needed. This also provides constant reinforcement of the purpose so that motivation does not flag.

The IIT-K ventilator task force was disbanded on 1 July 2020, and Nocca has now transitioned to a peacetime model where they are making rapid progress. Two experienced mentors – Rakesh Bhargava and Ajai Chowdhry – remain engaged using this five-point formula to ensure Nocca continues on the path of success during the post-pandemic period. Till September, they kept the momentum going through weekly meetings every Thursday. These calendarized interactions, that are now monthly, have been a huge source of motivation and direction for the Nocca founders. The mentors review the sales pipeline closely on an account-by-account basis to help Nocca plan and prioritize better. When Rakesh spotted that they were spending too much time focusing on big hospitals, he advised them, 'Don't chase them because they can afford expensive MNC ventilators. Why don't you go after these smaller nursing homes, especially in smaller cities where they have limited budgets?' Nocca's sales funnel in Chennai was looking good, but conversions were slow. By teaching them how to identify likely bottlenecks, Ajai helped them improve their sales forecasting.

Rakesh also made them acutely aware of the importance of measurement, 'Every task must have a measurable parameter. If you can't measure something, you can't change it.' Nocca is rapidly growing but struggling to hire talent fast enough. Rakesh's lessons have helped them identify the root cause of this problem by getting them to look at each step of the hiring process very closely. When they examined this closely, the founders discovered the real issue – they were meeting many candidates and making job offers, but candidates were dropping out after being made job offers. Sometimes, the candidates drop out because of a competing offer, but the founders are now focused on wooing the selected candidates and getting them excited about working at Nocca.

From the spectator stands, we are rooting for them to win big. If they grow well and succeed, it would be immensely satisfying for the entire task force. If we can replicate the ventilator project model at other startups, incubators and even in large companies, it would be a rewarding conclusion to our venture and a great contribution to the world of entrepreneurship and business in the post-Covid world.

KEY TAKEAWAYS

Missions can succeed even without a crisis.

- During times of crisis, people unite behind a common purpose to fight a perceived threat.
- But this kind of collaboration is possible in normal times too.
- The five-point formula to achieve this comprises an idea, a deadline, a champion, a safe environment and regular interactions to keep the group motivated.

STARTER KIT

STEP 1: The leader needs to create an environment where the sense of purpose, urgency and spirit of collaboration usually seen during times of crisis can be replicated during normal times. To get the ball rolling, the leader needs to take on and spell out the big problem and set a deadline for the problem to be resolved.

STEP 2: A small group of champion(s) must be assigned to work on the problem, who will then pull in other experts who are doers with good people skills, and are also passionate about solving the problem.

STEP 3: This group needs to work collaboratively, with openness, and without a tendency towards one-upmanship. Regular, planned meetings are important for building momentum and supporting each other. In the initial stages, it might even help to meet daily.

Notes

1. Feynman, Richard Phillips., Ralph Leighton, Bill Gates and Edward Hutchings. *'Surely You're Joking, Mr. Feynman!': Adventures of a Curious Character.* New York: W.W. Norton, 1985. It is an edited collection of reminiscences by the Nobel Prize-winning physicist Richard Feynman.
2. Viren Rasquinha's interview with the authors.

3. Ugra, Sharda. 'Junior World Cup Victory Puts Indian Hockey on Crossroads Again.' *India Today*, 5 November 2001. https://www.indiatoday.in/magazine/sport/story/20011105-junior-world-cup-victory-puts-indian-hockey-on-crossroads-again-774564-2001-11-05.
4. Dr Madhushree Nanda Agarwal's interview with the authors.
5. Anand Kripalu's interview with the authors.
6. Dr Leena Chatterjee's interview with the authors.
7. Shankkar Aiyar's interview with the authors.
8. Tiger Tyagarajan's interview with the authors.

Epilogue

Six months after the task force got disbanded, Nocca Robotics was renamed Noccarc Robotics. The ventilator product name, Noccarc, has now also become the company name. The child has become the parent.

There's a sparkling new website that reflects not just this name change, but also sharp thinking along two lines of business – solar and medtech. With demand picking up in both businesses, Nikhil and Harshit see the company clocking a revenue of ₹20 crore in the financial year 2020–21. Tushar is now in charge of new product development across both areas, and dreams of being an entrepreneur himself four years from now. Asim is thoroughly enjoying his post-retirement second innings as the chief operating officer and continues to find the Noccarc team 'simply super'.

The journey from 1 July – when the task force met for the last time – to the end of 2020 has expectedly been a rollercoaster ride for the Noccarc team. It would have been boring otherwise! The thrills have come from market acceptance. After a distributors' meeting on 8 July and the first commercial dispatch on 15 July to Petronet LNG, other orders came in quick succession.

Impressed by the ventilators, the distributors requested for a new product and the Noccarc team promptly agreed to do so. Based on High Flow Nasal Oxygen (HFNO) Therapy – one of the 'modes' in which the V310 ventilator operates – Noccarc designed an independent device, the H210 HFNO Therapy device. The product was launched on 22 August 2020.

At present, 265 Noccarc V310 and 140 Noccarc H210 devices are deployed in forty-eight cities and sixteen states in Covid centres, defence medical colleges and hospitals. From Pune's Ruby Hall Clinic and Goa Medical College in the west to Guwahati Medical College in the east, and from the district hospitals of Yamuna Nagar, Rohtak and Bhiwani in the north to Al Ameen Medical College and Hospital, Bijapur, in the south, these devices are making Noccarc's presence felt in small towns across the country as they were meant to.

Amidst this expansion spree, it rained heavily in Pune for three days and the Noccarc factory was flooded on 26 July. A hundred V310s were heroically evacuated in time. There was another minor blip when the founders and a few team members tested positive for Covid-19 on 13 October but work from home and a quick recovery meant there were no big setbacks.

Getting ready for international sales, the Noccarc team got their machines certified for IEC 60601-1-2, a higher level of certification than the IEC 60601-1 test required for DGHS's agnipariksha. The Noccarc V310 was certified on 11 August 2020 and the H210 on 24 August 2020.

Most importantly, doctors like the Noccarc products. As early as 8 August, Dr Prachee Sathe's team at Ruby Hall Clinic used the V310 to save the life of a patient in respiratory distress who was being shifted from another hospital into the clinic. Dr Awais Mahaldar of Mahaldar Children's Hospital, Bijapur (Karnataka), shared that he was really happy because the creators of V310 have focused on simplicity by 'identifying the essential [features] and eliminating the rest'.

Such positive response encouraged the team to invest in a new factory and office, which is almost six times bigger than the previous one. And yes, flood proof. They relocated on 20 October.

Both of us (authors) make it a point to call them often, partly to soak in the ongoing fun of their exciting journey, and partly to check if they need any help. And, of course, they continue to gain from the wisdom of Ajai, Rakesh and Saurabh through their monthly reviews.

Though Aditi felt lost for a while as she had got used to the daily fix of the noon Zoom call, she is now back to her regular routine as Program Manager at SIIC. She wishes we had created a short video recording the major task force milestones. This book should make her happy.

For Rahul Patel, working for the IIT Kanpur ventilator project was one of his top life experiences. After witnessing how 'the power of belief' can be used to solve any complex problem, he is busy celebrating the success of 'Abhivyakti 2020', the annual flagship event of SIIC, IIT Kanpur which he anchored in December.

As this strange year draws to an end, all the task force members walk away from 2020 with some great memories. Pavan recalls the speed at which everyone became friends, and being able to disagree without egos coming in the way. Rajesh echoes the same and adds how this was one of the most satisfying collaborative efforts of his life. Sanjay feels a sense of accomplishment having contributed to the nation's cause. Sanjiv was inspired to mentor yet another SIIC startup. The person who was impacted the most was Rakesh Bhargava. He had lost a dear family member in late 2019. Being in this task force – helping save lives – became his healing process.

Saurabh, Ajai and Padmaja routinely get involved with missionary zeal in projects that make a big impact for the startup ecosystem. At this point, they are in the thick of organizing the Startup India International Summit to celebrate the fifth anniversary of the Startup India initiative. The ventilator project remains a memorable and special project for them too.

For us, this has been a super-special experience. And a completely unexpected one at that. We feel lucky to have been part of something so meaningful and satisfying to alleviate the struggles of our frontline workers. And we feel privileged that we could work so closely with such a fantastic group of people. While the outcome in terms of a world-class product was great, the journey itself was very rewarding.

We are sure there are similar stories of struggle and triumph out there that will become a part of folklore when we look back at 2020 a few years down the line.

Srikant Sastri and Amitabha Bandyopadhyay
December 2020

Afterword

As I look back at this amazing experience, the first thing that strikes me is how quickly we eased into mission mode. Almost, it might appear, without sufficient thought. But this is the story of most innovative ventures: a heightened sense of urgency, the inability to wait for all the answers, and the confidence to deal with the inevitable twists and turns as they come.

Although we believe we may have accidentally discovered or even designed the new (and improved) Silicon Valley model, there are some prerequisites for it to work. These centre around four P's: people, passion, process and purpose. This phenomenal project worked primarily because of the people involved and their passion to succeed against all odds.

Amitabha committed himself 24/7 and his phenomenal team responded admirably to his call. Professor Karandikar backed us all the way and even joined many of our calls. Srikant interrupted his life to lead this effort round the clock. Ajai pulled in his former colleagues to solve the all-important supply chain problems, while the medical experts – Sanjay, Pawan and Sanjiv – were more hands-on doers than advisers. IAN, which had funded a different business plan, didn't blink an eye at Nocca's pivot, and Padmaja was on all the calls with me.

But what energized the entire task force were the young founders, Nikhil and Harshit, as if on steroids, their supreme confidence in themselves and their round-the-clock commitment to making it happen. All of us were aligned to our purpose. We were going to produce *a world-class ventilator at an affordable price within ninety days*. The final enabler was the process we put in place. The daily Zoom calls at noon for an hour or two were sacrosanct. Even if some members joined late or had other commitments, there was always an agenda, and everyone had their say. We had sub-groups for specific areas. Age and seniority played no role; equal respect was accorded to all, and thank goodness for that. The best suggestions often came from the youngest members. All of us had formidable experiences and reputations, many had never met before, yet there were no egos on display.

For me personally, this was one of my most enjoyable experiences, making me relive my memorable IIT student days. I was extremely encouraged that those we invited to the task force did not hesitate in saying yes. It was particularly heart-warming that many Indians in extremely senior positions in academia and industry overseas were more than happy to chip in with critical inputs and advice to the extent they could, without violating any of their confidentiality agreements with their employers. As they say, 'You can take an Indian out of India, but you can never take India out of an Indian.'

The level of cooperation and collaboration within the task force for almost three months was something I had never experienced in any group of senior industry experts, let alone our added diversity of domain experts, academics and enthusiastic youngsters. In fact, by the end of the project, many of us felt like we had known one another for ages!

Silicon Valley is unique. It works because the pieces of a problem and solutions lie in close geographical proximity. Passionate and aspirational entrepreneurs, mentors and advisers, angel investors and VCs are all barely an hour apart. Solutions are found in meetings and discussions in cafes, bars, homes and offices. The best and the brightest from around the world make their home in the Valley. There is no place in the world that can replicate this cocktail. But, during times such as a pandemic, all these advantages disappear. With our Nocca project, we replicated and actually improved on the Silicon Valley model as we captured the ambition and passion but transcended geographical limitations and accessed experts from around the world.

I believe this is a great model for all incubators and accelerators to use, especially the government ones. We used it for design and development and bringing to market a world-class product. However, the model can also be used for any part of a value chain, or the entire life cycle of a venture. The challenge will be to identify the right members for the relevant task force. Paradoxically, it should be easier for the government to attract right-minded mentors to help in what would be seen as a 'nation-building' activity, those who would not be as interested in remuneration as in perhaps recognition. Non-government incubators may have to consider some form of ESOPs (employee stock ownerships).

Perhaps a national framework can be created for chosen domains where we wish to focus (healthcare is just one). This can become a powerful tool to help drive India's 'Atmanirbhar' agenda. I have suggested this model to some of the government entities involved in innovation and support of incubators and accelerators.

This exciting story was also made possible by some external factors. It was Prime Minister Narendra Modi's championing of the startup movement that made India the world's third-largest hub. It was also his clarion call to find local solutions to Covid-19 that inspired Nikhil and Harshit to attempt the impossible. We received massive support from various government agencies. Dr K. VijayRaghavan, the principal scientific advisor to the government, was a constant source of encouragement and inspiration. Invest India helped us with our supply chain issues in sourcing components, and state and municipal corporations helped the company operate in Covid times. BIRAC and DST were extremely supportive in helping fund some of the R&D. The private sector chipped in too – Standard Chartered Bank, ICICI Securities, Infoedge, ANSYS and ACT (a special-purpose entity set up by leading VCs solely for providing financial support to Covid-focused ventures).

The only disappointment in this otherwise exciting and enjoyable fairy tale was the government's centralized procurement process for ventilators. With the government purchasing around 60,000 ventilators, more than all private procurement put together, we had hoped that at least 25% of this quantity would be spread across startups like Nocca, where the product was certified by government agencies as meeting all specifications and had been installed, accepted and certified by the country's leading private hospitals. Had that happened, it would have given Nocca an immediate launch pad into the global market. Nocca seemed like such an ideal candidate – a startup founded by IIT grads, incubated and strongly supported by IIT Kanpur and its incubator, backed by leading Indian industry lights in India and overseas, and delivering from scratch a world-class, sophisticated ICU-use ventilator in ninety days, something which normally takes two to three years!

Unfortunately, that didn't happen. Nocca and India missed a great opportunity here.

I believe that government procurement, especially in India, where it is the largest buyer of most products, should be used to encourage and give a strong positive signal to Indian entrepreneurs and academic institutions that create innovations furthering the 'Atmanirbhar Programme'. Most global winners succeed by first scaling in their own markets. I would urge the government to step in and help unleash our world-class startups on the global market. Nocca, of course, will still be a global success story, though it might take a bit longer. Even as I write this piece, Nocca has already moved on to its next world-class product, one which India needs in large numbers: the HFNO machine.

Saurabh Srivastava
September 2020

(Saurabh Srivastava has been a serial entrepreneur, and an angel and VC investor. He has founded and chaired NASSCOM, TiE, IVCA and IAN. Among many awards, he has received an award from Prime Minister Narendra Modi for his contribution to the Indian IT industry, and a Padma Shri for his contribution towards building the Indian entrepreneurial ecosystem. He is a Distinguished Alumnus of IIT Kanpur, a member of the board of FIRST, IIT Kanpur's incubator, and has been an early mentor to Nocca before they raised capital from IAN.)

Acknowledgements

Those who made the book happen

Rachna Kalra: friend, publishing veteran and advisor who convinced Kanishka Gupta that he should be our literary agent

Kanishka Gupta: literary agent and consultant; his pace and drive are phenomenal

Teesta Guha Sarkar: our editor at Pan Macmillan India who graciously took us first-timers under her wings to turn our raw thinking into a reasonably sculpted product

Amish Mulmi: he had the unenviable task of bringing chalk and cheese together, of bringing consistency across the very different writing styles that both of us have

Seema Choudhary: chipped in with ideas to reach out to Kanishka

Those who contributed content for the book

Dr Abhay Karandikar (Foreword)

Saurabh Srivastava (Afterword)

Dr Prachee Sathe ('The Ventilator Primer')

Dr Deepak Padmanbhan ('The Ventilator Primer')

Tushar Agarwal ('The Ventilator Primer')

Aditi Kumar ('Pennies from Heaven')

Those who gave time for interviews

Government: Ajay Bisaria, Rahul Chhabra, Chandrima Sinha

Science and technology ecosystem: Dr Ashutosh Sharma, Dr Renu Swarup, Dr Anita Gupta, Dr Manish Diwan, Dr Ashwini Nangia, Anil Jauhari, M. G. Sathyendra, Dr V. Premnath

Academia: Dr Vijay Kumar, Dr Gautam Ahuja, Dr Gita Johar, Dr Jaideep Srivastava, Dr Ananth Raman, Dr Rishikesha Krishnan, Dr Leena Chatterjee, Dr Madhushree Nanda Agarwal

Industry and business leaders: Sanjeev Maddila, Dr Pramath Raj Sinha, Anand Kripalu, Anil Kumar Sharma, Nirmal Kishore Jain, Atul Mishra, Chirag Gala, Tapesh Sinha, Tiger Tyagrajan, Rishad Tobaccowala, Vipin Sondhi, Sriram Sankar, Sanjeev Maddila, Shreyasi Singh, Sunil Singh

Doctors: Sujata Mishra, A. V. S. Ravi, Sunil Nandwani, Prachee Sathe, C. S. Pant

Medical technology: Yashdeep Kumar, V. Raja

Sports and entertainment: Viren Rasquinha, Harsha Bhogle, Imtiaz Ali

Startup ecosystem: Vijaya Kumar Ivaturi, Dr Subhrangshu Sanyal, Nikhil Agarwal, Sandip Patil

Others: Shankkar Aiyar

The ones who read the manuscript in whole or in part and/or advised us first-time authors

Shreyasi Singh, Rishad Tobaccowala, Shankkar Aiyar, Sudha Sastri, Siddharth Sastri, Nishtha Jain, Sachin Sastri, Vijay Gokhale, Kanika Mathur, Dr Deepak Padmanabhan

Those who were generous with their praise and endorsed the book

Dr K. VijayRaghavan, Gopal Vittal, Dr Pramath Raj Sinha, Samir Arora, Sanjiv Puri, Ramesh Ramadurai, Suresh Shankar, Dinesh Agarwal, Geetika Dayal, Navyug Mohnot, Shankkar Aiyar, Rishad Tobaccowala, Dr Anju Seth, Venky Shankar, Dr Ashwini Kumar Nangia, Dr Ashish Diwan, Dr Gourdas Choudhuri, Amith Prabhu, Kandy Anand, Rohit Thakur

Organizations and people across the world who helped the IIT Kanpur ventilator task force

Government: Cabinet Secretariat, Principal Scientific Advisor to the Government of India, the Ministry of Electronics and Information Technology, Invest India, Ministry of Civil Aviation, Indian High Commission at Singapore, Venugopal Reddy (IAS), Dr Rubal Agarwal (IAS)

Science and technology ecosystem: Dr Ashutosh Sharma, Dr Anita Gupta, Dr Renu Swarup, Dr Manish Diwan, CAWACH – DST

Doctors: Prachee Sathe, Deepak Padmanabhan, Govind Rajan, Prakash Keshaviah, Dileep Raman

Medical technology: Yashdeep Kumar

CSR donors: ANSYS, Standard Chartered, ICICI Securities, ACT, Infoedge, Marico Foundation

Industry and business leaders: Tapesh Sinha, Sudhir Mehta

Manufacturers: Chirag Gala

Former IIT Kanpur students: Abhishek Kulkarni, Elle Atma Vidya Prakash, Kshitij Jaggi, Kumar Shivang, Rishabh Sahu

Good samaritans in India: The members of the 'Caring Indians' Twitter group, especially Dr Santosh Ansumali, Dr Aloke Kumar, Mr Manish Mundra, among others

Good samaritans in Singapore: Shailendra Gupta, Kanika Mathur, Anurag Srivastava, Sanjiv Aiyar, Siddharth Harlalka

The ventilator task force

All of whom feature throughout this book, plus a few others who came in for short durations: Madhav Sikka and Sanat Mondal from IAN, Vineet Kumar from Nocca Robotics

Our families

Our families who first watched us get fully consumed by the ventilator project for ninety days, and then again as we became engrossed in writing this book, while they coped with the lockdown on their own, without our company. Special thanks to Sudha Sastri for suggesting the idea for this book.